QUIZZES AND QUESTIONS FOR NURSES

Book B. Surgical Nursing and Geriatric Nursing

QUIZZES AND QUESTIONS
for Nurses

Book B. Surgical Nursing and Geriatric Nursing

E. J. HULL BA, SRN, RNT
Formerly Principal Tutor, Luton and Dunstable Hospital

B. J. ISAACS SRN, Part 1 CMB, RNT
Director of Nurse Education, Bedfordshire Area Health
Authority ; Member of the Examining Board of the General
Nursing Council for England and Wales

BAILLIÈRE TINDALL
LONDON

A BAILLIÈRE TINDALL book published by
Cassell & Collier Macmillan Publishers Ltd
35 Red Lion Square, London WC1R 4SG
and at Sydney, Auckland, Toronto, Johannesburg
an affiliate of
Macmillan Publishing Co. Inc.
New York

First published 1976

SBN 0 7020 0599 1

Printed by The Whitefriars Press Ltd,
London and Tonbridge

CONTENTS

PREFACE

The ideas behind *Quizzes and Questions for Nurses* are similar to those underlying our previous series, *Do-It-Yourself Revision for Nurses*. It aims to provide a plan of revision, based on examination questions and 'model answers'.

In the present book, however, the majority of the questions are taken from papers set for the assessment of pupil nurses; but, as they all deal with topics and situations met with by *all* nurses, we hope that they will be helpful not only to pupils but to student nurses as well, especially in the earlier part of their training. Although the scope of knowledge is somewhat less than in the former books, we hope we have set a standard acceptable for any learner engaged in basic nurse training.

We have somewhat modified our plan in the 'revision' part of each chapter. Instead of a simple list of 'Points to revise' which we gave in our former books, the revision takes the form of a quiz, with answers and explanations, covering all the material needed for answering a question. We hope in this way to give learners more guidance in their revision.

After the revision quiz and explanations comes the question, to be answered so far as possible under examination conditions; and this is followed by a 'model answer' with a marking scheme by which the learner can mark her own work. The method of using the book is explained in more detail in the Introduction.

We hope that those who use the books will find this method interesting, helpful and encouraging.

February 1976

E. J. Hull
B. J. Isaacs

Introduction

TO THE STUDENT—HOW TO USE THIS BOOK

DO NOT SKIP THE INTRODUCTION: it shows you how to get most help from the book.

(a) You will see that there are two *main sections* in the book: Surgical Nursing and Geriatric Nursing. The book has been written to help you to *revise*; so you should only tackle chapters in a section when you have already had the right type of experience, i.e. if you have worked on a geriatric ward, but not on a surgical one, start with the 'Geriatric Nursing' section, and leave the 'Surgical Nursing' until you have been on a surgical ward.

(b) There are two questions on 'First Aid and Emergencies' at the end of the book. You may be able to answer these whatever experience you have had.

(c) Even if you have not been nursing for very long, you have had *some* experience, and should be able to answer some of the questions. So start revising in good time, and don't leave all your revision until the last weeks before your examination.

(d) Each chapter in the book starts with a lot of very short 'revision questions'—a *quiz* covering some part of the syllabus. You must answer these questions FIRST. You can do them on your own or discuss them in a group. In either case, WRITE DOWN the answers. In some of the questions you simply have to choose the right answer from several alternatives; in others you have to write a few words or draw a diagram. When you have finished this, find the correct answers on the next page. There is also some explanation of the answers. You correct your own answers and see how well you have scored. The idea is to help you to recall what you do know and show you what you don't.
    NOW, do any more revision you need, and fill in gaps you have found in your knowledge.

(e) So far, so good. But in your examinations, as you know, you do not have a quiz with very short answers, but have to write longer answers, each taking about 40 minutes. So the second part of each chapter gives you practice in this. There is a question to be answered under examination conditions, which you should answer without looking back or using books, allowing yourself not more than 40 minutes. Needless to say, the quiz and the question do not *have* to be done on the same day.

(f) When you have written your answer (NOT before), you turn over to the next page. Here there is a 'model answer', with a scheme for making your own work. You should do this as soon as possible.

The first section contains a quiz and a question for practice, with some advice on marking.

NOW start on the quiz on the next page.

Practice Quiz and Question

1 FUNCTIONS OF THE SKIN; CARE OF THE SKIN, NAILS AND HAIR

REVISION QUIZ

1. Here is a diagram of the skin. Name the structures in the skin labelled A to E.

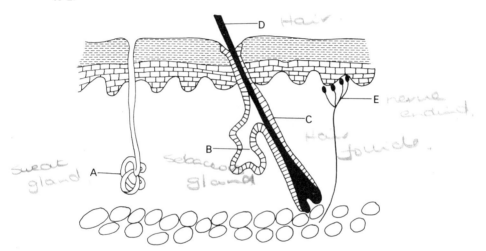

In each of questions 2–10 there is only ONE correct answer. You have to choose this; so write A, B or C, etc., ONLY.

2. Is the outer layer of the skin, composed of many layers of cells

   A. the epidermis   B. the dermis
   C. the subcutaneous layer

3. Is the entry of bacteria prevented by

   A. the epidermis   B. the dermis
   C. the subcutaneous layer

4. Is the secretion which prevents the skin becoming cracked called

   A. sweat   B. sebum
   C. ergosterol   D. mucus

5. Is the skin

    A. porous   B. waterproof

6. Is the body protected from sunburn by

    A. the thickness of the skin   B. sebum
    C. ergosterol   D. pigment in the skin

7. Sweat helps to cool the body. Does it do this by

    A. removing waste products   B. radiation
    C. evaporation

8. When the body is hot, do the small blood vessels in the skin

    A. dilate   B. constrict
    C. move nearer to the surface   D. move away from the surface

9. Is the effect of sunlight (or ultraviolet light) on the skin

    A. to produce vitamin A   B. to produce vitamin C
    C. to produce vitamin D   D. to produce ergosterol

10. You have a bedridden patient. Which of the following do you consider
    the *most important* in the care of her pressure areas

    A. massaging them
    B. applying barrier cream
    C. supplying her with an air ring
    D. supplying her with a sheepskin to lie on
    E. changing her position frequently

Now WRITE answers to the following questions.

11. List all the pressure areas. *Skull, ears, zygomatic bone*
    elbow sacral greater
    trocanter, knee, heels
    ankle

12. List areas where two skin surfaces meet.

Now correct your answers from the notes on pages 5 and 6.

4

ANSWERS AND NOTES ON REVISION QUIZ

1. A = sweat gland   B = sebaceous gland
    C = hair follicle   D = hair
    E = nerve ending

    Count ONE mark for each structure correctly named (= 5 marks).

    These parts of the skin all play a part in its functions. The nerve endings are sensitive to touch, pain, heat and cold.

For questions 2–10 count TWO marks for each correct answer.

Correct answer

2. A. The *epidermis* is the outer layer; the dermis is the next, fibrous layer which supports blood vessels, sweat glands, etc.; subcutaneous layer is below it, consisting largely of fat.

3. A. So long as the skin is not broken, the tightly packed cells of the epidermis prevent bacteria from entering.

4. B. Sebum is the oily secretion made by sebaceous glands. As you see in the diagram, they pour sebum into the hair follicles. It keeps hair and skin slightly oily and prevents cracking.

5. B. Skin is waterproof. The outside cells are dry. This prevents bacteria entering and prevents loss of fluid from the tissues underneath.

6. D. Pigment (colouring matter) in the skin protects against ultraviolet rays in sunlight. More pigment develops if the skin is exposed to the sun.

7. C. Sweat *evaporates*. This takes heat from the skin.

8. A. Small blood vessels in the skin dilate (enlarge) when the body is hot, so that heat is lost from them into the air outside by radiation.

    Together the sweat glands and blood vessels help to regulate the body temperature. If the body is cold, less sweat is produced and the blood vessels constrict (or become narrower).

9. C. *Vitamin D* is produced from the fatty substance ergosterol by the action of sunlight.

10. E. Changing the patient's position is probably the *most* important way of preventing pressure on these areas, though of course it is also important to keep skin dry and free from injury and pressure in other ways.

For questions 11 and 12 count mark as indicated.

11. Sacrum, heels, shoulder blades, spine, hips, elbows, between knees (1 mark for each = 7 marks).

12. Under breasts; axillae; groins; between toes (1 mark for each = 4 marks).

Note to Student. As you will see, part (b) of the question on the opposite page is very straightforward; so we have only given you three questions about care of the skin in the quiz. These three questions are just to remind you of some of the detail you should put in—and that ways of relieving pressure are all part of care of the *skin*.

Maximum Total = 34 marks.

Your score will show you how well you have done. Do any more revision which you think you need BEFORE attempting the question on the page opposite.

QUESTION

Without looking back or consulting any book, write the answer to the question on this page. You should not take more than 40 minutes to plan and write your answer.

(a) Give a brief account of the main functions of the skin.
(b) Describe the care which you would give to the skin, nails and hair of a patient who is bedridden.

READ THE QUESTION CAREFULLY. Underline words you think are important, such as 'functions'. This will remind you that the question does *not* ask you to describe the *structure* of the skin. It avoids your wasting time writing what examiners call 'irrelevant matter'.

When you have finished your answer, and not before, turn over and correct it by the 'model answer' overleaf.

MODEL ANSWER

Note on correcting answers. You will have found it quite easy to correct the *quiz*; but correcting answers to questions needs more judgement. This is because no two people will write an answer in exactly the same words, or put the different points in quite the same order. So look for the *points*, not exact words. If you have the same point in different words, count the marks for it. Examples of different ways of saying the same thing are given in brackets, thus: (*or . . .*). But there will still be other ways in which you may have made the same point.

Now correct your work by this *model answer.*

(a) *Functions of the skin* (40 marks)

Unbroken skin prevents the entry of bacteria (*or* germs) (5). It also protects the tissues underneath from injury (4), and prevents loss of fluid from the tissues (2). Pigment in the skin (*or* melanin) (2) prevents burning by the sun (*or* by ultraviolet rays *or* from radiation) (2).

The skin helps to regulate body temperature (4) by producing sweat (2). This causes loss of heat by evaporation (1). Heat is also lost from blood vessels in the skin (2), which dilate when the body is hot (1). When the body is cold, the skin produces less sweat (1) and the blood vessels constrict (*or* narrow) (1). Fat in the deep layers of the skin helps to keep the body warm (*or* prevents loss of heat, *or* insulates the body) (1).

Vitamin D (2) is formed by the action of sunlight (*or* ultraviolet rays) (2) on the deep layers of the skin (1).

The skin contains nerve endings (*or* is a sense organ) (4) sensitive to sensations of touch (1), pain (1) and temperature (1).

(b) *Care of skin, nails and hair of a bedridden patient* (60 marks)

The patient must have regular bed baths (3). The skin must be kept dry (2), especially under the breasts (1), in the axillae (1) and groins (1) and between the toes (1) (*or* 4 marks for just saying 'where two skin surfaces meet'). Talcum powder should be used for these (2).

Night clothes and bed-linen must be changed regularly (1), and whenever they become soiled or wet (2). Sheets must be kept free from wrinkles (1) and crumbs (1).

Skin over the pressure areas needs special care (2), especially if the patient is thin (2). Areas which may become red and sore are sacrum (1), heels (1), shoulder blades (1), spine (1), hips (1), elbows (1) and between the knees (1). The patient's position should be changed every 4 hours (3), or more frequently if she cannot move herself (2). Bed cradles can be used to keep bedclothes from pressing on the feet or paralysed limbs (2), and a pillow with waterproof cover between the kees will prevent sores on these (2). Sheepskins, air rings, sorbo rings, heel pads of sponge rubber and ripple mattresses can be used (count 2 marks each for any three of these = 6 marks). Whenever the patient is moved, pressure areas are washed and dried (2) and powdered (1). If the patient is incontinent, barrier cream (*or* examples such as zinc and castor oil ointment, Thovaline, etc.) is applied (3).

The fingernails should be kept clean and short (2), and the cuticles pushed down (1). Toe nails are cut straight across (1). If they are very hard and horny, a chiropodist should attend to them (2).

Hair should be kept brushed and combed (2). Long hair should be arranged so that it does not get tangled (2). If possible, regular visits from a hairdresser should be arranged for a woman so that her hair can be washed and set (2).

Now add up your marks. It is a good idea to keep a record of your marks for each question. You will find that they improve as you get more practice in writing answers. If you do get poor marks for a question, you will learn quite a lot as you correct your answer. You can prove this if you try the same question again after a few weeks. For a pass, you should aim at getting 55 to 60 marks out of 100 on a question. If you get 70, you are probably doing very well. In an examination, hardly anybody ever writes a *perfect* answer!

Surgical Nursing

2 ACUTE APPENDICITIS: PREOPERATIVE PREPARATION

REVISION QUIZ

In questions 1 and 2 there is only ONE correct answer. You have to choose this; so write A, B or C, etc., ONLY.

1. A patient is under age, and his parents cannot be contacted to sign a form of consent for an urgent operation. Should the nurse in charge

    A. ask him to sign the form himself
    B. send him to the theatre with a note explaining why the form is not signed
    C. report the facts to the surgeon before preparing the patient for theatre

2. A patient is under observation while waiting to have an operation for appendicitis. Which of the following would be the most urgent to report

    A. a rise in the pulse rate
    B. a fall in the pulse rate
    C. a rise in temperature
    D. a fall in temperature

Now WRITE answers to the following questions.

3. List the routine observations which a nurse should make when a patient is admitted for operation.

4. List the nurse's responsibilities in preparing a patient for an abdominal operation with regard to

    (a) relieving the patient's anxiety
    (b) lessening the risk of the wound becoming infected
    (c) making sure that the right patient has the right operation
    (d) ensuring that the surgeon and anaesthetist have all the information which they need

Now correct your answers from the notes on page 12.

ANSWERS AND NOTES ON REVISION QUIZ

For questions 1 and 2 count TWO marks for each correct answer.

Correct answer

1. C. The surgeon will have to decide whether the patient is old or responsible enough to sign his own consent form.

2. A. Rise in pulse rate, in a patient with an acute abdominal condition, might mean perforation and peritonitis.

For questions 3 and 4 count marks as indicated.

3. Testing urine for abnormalities (2)
   Temperature (1), pulse (1), respiration (1)
   Observations of anything which might lead to postoperative complications, e.g. a cough or cold (2), septic spots (2).

4. (a) Answering questions about his preparation for theatre, which may worry him or seem strange (2); explaining effects his premedication (2); reassuring by having cheerful and sympathetic manner (2).
   (b) Shaving of the abdomen (2) and pubic area (2); making sure area is clean (2), especially umbilicus (2); reporting any septic spots, etc. (2).
   (c) Attaching identity bracelet (2), filled in with full name (2), hospital number (2) and ward (2); seeing that right notes accompany patient to theatre (2).
   (d) Seeing that notes are in order and correctly filled in (2); writing time of premedication on drug sheet (2), and result of urine test on notes (2).

Maximum Total = 45 marks.

Your score will show you how well you have done. Do any more revision which you think you need BEFORE attempting the question on the page opposite.

QUESTION

Without looking back or consulting any book, write the answer to the question on this page. You should not take more than 40 minutes to plan and write your answer.

A youth of 17 years is admitted to the ward as an emergency with acute appendicitis.

(a) Describe how you would prepare the patient for operation.
(b) What would you observe and report on the patient before he is taken to the operating theatre?

When you have finished your answer, and not before, turn over and correct it by the 'model answer' overleaf.

13

MODEL ANSWER

(a) *Preparation for operation* (70 marks)

I would screen the bed (2) and give the patient a urinal and ask him to pass urine so that a specimen could be tested (3).

I would then explain that I was going to get him ready to go to theatre (2). I would try to reassure him (1), telling him that he will have an injection which will relieve his pain (2) and that he will probably be asleep when he goes to the theatre (2).

I would shave his abdomen (3) and pubic area (3), and wash and dry them, making sure that he was clean (2), especially his umbilicus (2). If he was really dirty he would need a bed bath (3).

I would dress him in an operation gown (2) and socks (1), and cover his hair, which might be long, with a cap or triangular bandage (3). I would explain that the reason for all this was that we had to make sure no germs could get into his wound (3).

I would fill in an identity bracelet (4) with his full name (2), hospital number (2) and ward (2), and attach it to his ankle or wrist (2).

Next his premedication would be checked (3) and given half to three-quarters of an hour before he was due to go to the theatre (3). He would be left to sleep if possible until the theatre trolley arrived (2).

I would sign the prescription for the premedication on his drug sheet as having been given (3). I would check that a form for consent to operation had been signed by his parents (3); as if for any reason they could not be contacted the surgeon must be told immediately (2). I would make sure his notes were complete (3) and take them with me when I escorted him to the theatre (2).

If some time had elapsed since he passed urine, he should be given a urinal again before going to the theatre, so that his bladder was empty (3).

(b) *Observations* (30 marks)

I would test the patient's urine as soon as possible after his admission (4), and report to the nurse in charge whether or not it contained abnormalities (2). The result would be written on the patient's notes before he went to theatre (2).

His temperature, pulse and respiration and blood pressure would be taken and reported (4), and entered on his chart (2). If he were not going to theatre immediately, I would keep a quarter-hourly record of his pulse rate (2), and report if this were rising (2).

I would report it if I noticed any septic spots on the patient's body (2); or if he had a cough or cold (2); if he vomited (2), or if his pain seemed to be getting worse (2).

It would be very important to report if he had not passed urine before going to the theatre (4).

14

Surgical Nursing

3 POSTOPERATIVE COMPLICATIONS AND DISCOMFORTS

REVISION QUIZ

1. Which TWO of the following complications are most likely to occur within the first two days after an abdominal operation

    A. wound infection
    C. deep venous thrombosis
    E. pulmonary embolus

    B. chest infection
    D. paralytic ileus
    F. pelvic abscess

2. Say whether each of the following statements is TRUE or FALSE.

    (a) A patient with a paralytic ileus does not vomit. — false.
    (b) A patient with a paralytic ileus becomes dehydrated. — True.
    (c) Peritonitis is a cause of paralytic ileus. — false.
    (d) A pulmonary embolus is the result of a chest infection. — false

3. List ways in which a patient's progress after operation may be hindered

    (a) if he is a heavy smoker
    (b) if he is obese

4. List nursing measures which can be taken after an abdominal operation

    (a) to help a patient who cannot pass urine
    (b) to avoid chest complications
    (c) to lessen pain
    (d) to relieve flatulence

Now correct your answers from the notes on page 16.

1.   B. and D. Chest infection and paralytic ileus (2 marks each = 4). The other complications mentioned are likely to occur later than two days after an operation.

2.   (a) FALSE (2). He does vomit unless the fluid is aspirated through a nasogastric tube. In paralytic ileus there is no peristalsis, so fluid and flatus collect in the intestine and stomach, as they cannot pass down.
     (b) TRUE (2). He is dehydrated because fluid cannot be absorbed.
     (c) TRUE (2). Peritonitis is the chief cause of paralytic ileus. To some extent it is also caused by the handling of the intestines during the operation.
     (d) FALSE (2). Pulmonary embolus is not the result of chest infection. It is caused by deep venous thrombosis; a piece of clot from the leg veins travels to the heart and then on to the lungs.

3.   (a) A heavy smoker is more liable to chest infection (2).
     (b) An obese patient is also more liable to chest infection (2). He may find it harder to move about, and so be more liable to thrombosis in the leg veins (2). He is also more likely to burst his stitches, especially if he has a cough (2).

4.   (a) It is easier to pass urine in a more normal position; so getting a man to stand out of bed with a urinal (2) or a woman onto a commode (2) may help. Running taps also sometimes help psychologically (2).
     (b) Encourage the patient to cough (2) to get rid of plugs of mucus which block the bronchi. Also movement helps his breathing (2).
     (c) Make sure the patient is given his postoperative analgesic as soon as he is round from the anaesthetic (2); show him how to hold his abdomen when he coughs (2).
     (d) Movement and getting out of bed help a patient to pass wind (2). A flatus tube can be passed (2).

Maximum Total = 38 marks.

Your score will show you how well you have done. Do any more revision which you think you need BEFORE attempting the question on the page opposite.

QUESTION

Without looking back or consulting any book, write the answer to the question on this page. You should not take more than 40 minutes to plan and write your answer.

A patient had a simple abdominal operation two days ago.

    (a) What are the possible reasons for this patient not making the expected progress after this operation?
    (b) What discomforts may occur postoperatively and how can the nurse help to deal with these discomforts?

When you have finished your answer, and not before, turn over and correct it by the 'model answer' overleaf.

MODEL ANSWER

(a) *Reasons for lack of progress* (50 marks)

The patient might have a paralytic ileus (4), due to handling of the intestines during the operation (1) or to peritonitis (2). He would then become dehydrated (2), because fluid collects in intestine and stomach and is vomited (1) or has to be aspirated (1). Flatus also cannot pass down and causes discomfort (2).

Lack of progress might also be due to a chest infection (5). This may be partly due to the anaesthetic (2). It is more likely if the patient is a heavy smoker (2), or is obese (2); or if he had a cold before the operation (2). It is also more likely if he is reluctant after the operation to cough (2) or move (1).

Poor physical condition before the operation might affect his progress (1), for example anaemia (2) or a chest complaint (2), although these would normally be dealt with preoperatively (1).

His mental outlook might affect progress (2), making him uncooperative (1), so that he would not take enough fluid (2) or help himself by moving (2).

An obese patient with a cough (3) might burst his stitches (3), necessitating a return to the theatre (2).

(b) *Postoperative discomforts* (50 marks)

There will be some pain and soreness of the wound (3). The nurse must see that the patient is given the pain-relieving drug ordered as soon as he needs it (2). She should also show him how to hold his abdomen when he coughs to prevent pain (2).

He may feel hot and uncomfortable on return from the threatre (3), and have a dry mouth (3). As soon as possible he should have his face and hands sponged (2), and be changed into his own night clothes (2), and be given a mouthwash or helped to clean his teeth (2). His position must be changed when necessary so that he is comfortable (1).

A patient may have difficulty in passing urine (3), because of being afraid to relax (1) and of being in an unnatural position (1). With screens round the bed (1), a man should be helped to stand out of bed with a urinal (2). A woman may find it easier to use a commode than a bed-pan (2). A running tap near by may help psychologically (1).

Postoperative vomiting may occur (3). The nurse should give the patient only sips of water when he first recovers from the anaesthetic (2). If he vomits, she can hold his forehead (2), wipe away any vomit from his face and neck (2), and remove the vomit immediately (2).

He may suffer from a lot of flatus (3). Helping him to move or get up may help him to pass it (2). If necessary the nurse can pass a flatus tube (3).

18

Surgical Nursing

4 HAEMORRHOIDS

In each of the following questions there is only ONE correct answer. You have to choose this; so write A, B or C, etc., ONLY.

1. Patients who have haemorrhoids often complain of tiredness. Is this because

    A. they are unable to sleep because of the pain
    B. they are unable to have a proper diet
    C. they are becoming increasingly anaemic

2. Are the stools of a patient with haemorrhoids likely to be

    A. relaxed   B. constipated   C. normal

3. Are the stools likely to contain

    A. blood and mucus   B. mucus only   C. blood only

4. Will the patient complain of

    A. constant pain   B. pain on defaecation
    C. colicky pain   D. pain on passing urine

5. Which is the most likely postoperative complication after haemorrhoidectomy? Is it

    A. retention of urine   B. diarrhoea
    C. abdominal pain

Now WRITE the answer to the following question.

6. A patient has had a haemorrhoidectomy. List the main points of any postoperative care you have seen used

    (a) to the operation area
    (b) for the bowels
    (c) regarding his diet

Now correct your answers from the notes on page 21.

ANSWERS AND NOTES ON REVISION QUIZ

For questions 1–5, count TWO marks for each correct answer.

Correct answer

1. C. This condition is one of the commonest causes of anaemia, because of the frequent small amounts of blood lost from the rectum.

2. B. Patients with haemorrhoids become constipated because they are afraid of the pain; as constipation is a *cause* of haemorrhoids, a 'vicious circle' is set up.

3. C. Mucus is passed in stools in ulcerative conditions of the colon; haemorrhoids are a local abnormality causing bleeding.

4. B.

5. A. It is good to remember this—if a patient has not passed urine by 12 hours after operation, it should be reported.

For question 6 count marks as indicated.

6. (a) EITHER: a wick of petroleum jelly gauze (or tulle gras) is inserted into the anus at operation. This says in until the patient takes a saline bath, usually on the following day. After the bath, a small tulle gras wick is reinserted and this is repeated once or twice daily until the area is healed—after about 7–10 days. Covered with a sterile dressing. A doctor may perform a rectal examination on the 7th postoperative day. The patient may have to dilate the anus with a metal dilator daily until seen in the out-patients' clinic.

    OR: a rubber drain, surrounded by petroleum jelly gauze is inserted at operation. On the third postoperative day, an olive oil enema is given through the tube which then is easily removed. After the enema, a saline bath is taken and repeated daily or twice daily.

    Count TEN marks for either method. If you have seen another method, discuss with your colleagues.

    (b) (c) EITHER: a normal diet is given so that a bulky stool is produced; some surgeons order extra roughage for this purpose. The stool helps to dilate the anus.

21

OR: a low-residue diet is ordered to confine the bowels for 2—3 days. Then an olive oil enema, followed by an enema saponis (*or* disposable enema) is given. Paraffin emulsion is given once or twice daily after the second postoperative day to keep the stools soft and make defaecation less painful.

Count TEN marks for either method.

The patient will be advised about his diet before discharge (2).

Maximum Total = 32 marks.

Your score will show you how well you have done. Do any more revision which you think you need BEFORE attempting the question on the page opposite.

QUESTION

Without looking back or consulting any book, write the answer to the question on this page. You should not take more than 40 minutes to plan and write your answer.

A middle-aged patient is admitted for haemorrhoidectomy.

    (a) What are haemorrhoids?
    (b) What symptoms might the patient have complained of before admission?
    (c) Describe the care needed postoperatively until the day of discharge.

When you have finished your answer, and not before, turn over and correct it by the 'model answer' overleaf.

MODEL ANSWER

(a) *What are haemorrhoids?* (10 marks)

Dilated (2) varicosed (*or* twisted and swollen) (4) veins in the region of the anus (4).

(b) *Symptoms before admission* (20 marks)

Bleeding on passing faeces (5). It would be bright red blood (2), severe or slight (1).
    Pain on defaecation, often very severe (3), especially when constipated (1). Constipation due to fear of pain (2).
    The patient feels tired (1) and looks pale due to anaemia (2).
    Some patients complain of a 'lump' near the anus if the piles prolapse (3).

(c) *Postoperative care* (70 marks)

While unconscious, the patient is placed in the semiprone position with his head to one side (3) so that a clear airway can be maintained (3). A nurse should stay with him until he is conscious (3).
    His pulse should be recorded half-hourly and any rise reported at once (3). His dressing should be inspected frequently for excessive bleeding (3).
    When conscious, he can have his hands and face washed and his operation gown replaced by his own pyjamas (3). If his condition is satisfactory, he should be sat up on an air-ring or sheepskin for comfort (3). The nurse must make sure his dressing is in place and repacks it if necessary (2).
    A pain-relieving drug should be given as ordered by the doctor (3).
    If there is no vomiting, sips of water can be given (2) and the amount recorded on a fluid balance chart (1). It should be reported if the patient does not pass urine after 12 hours (4); he may be allowed out of bed with help to make this easier for him (3).
    Analgesics may be required four- to six-hourly for the first few days (3).
    On the day after operation he is allowed up (1) with assistance and should be given a saline bath (3). After this a fresh dressing is applied according to the surgeon's wishes (*or* you may describe the method you have seen, such as a wick of eusol and paraffin soaked gauze inserted gently into the anus) (3).
    He is allowed to eat as he wishes (2) (*or* you may have said that a low-residue diet is given) or according to instructions (1).
    On the second evening a mild aperient may be ordered (*or* you can specify Milpar, Senakot or any you have used) (2) and this may be given once or twice each day following (1).
    If the patient does not have his bowels open by the third postoperative day, an olive oil enema may be ordered, followed by a soap and water (*or*

disposable) enema (2). The result should be reported and the nurse should look for any bleeding (2). This is followed by a saline bath and fresh dressing (2).

Baths and dressings are given daily (1).

On the seventh day the surgeon may perform a rectal examination to see if the area has healed (2); the nurse prepares the tray for this (1), puts the patient into the left lateral position (1) and stays to comfort and reassure him that it will not be too painful (1).

The patient will probably be allowed home after this (2). Advice is given him about his diet and medicines (2). An appointment is given him to attend the out-patients' clinic at a later date (2).

Surgical Nursing

5 WOUND INFECTION AND ITS PREVENTION

REVISION QUIZ

In each of questions 1–6 there is only ONE correct answer. You have to choose this; so write A, B or C, etc., ONLY.

1. Which of the following is the best arrangement of work on a surgical ward

   A. bedmaking and cleaning, then bed baths, dressings and medicines going on at the same time, to finish by lunch time
   B. bedmaking and cleaning, followed by medicines and other treatments; then dressings; with bed baths later in the day
   C. cleaning, followed by bed baths and bedmaking; then dressings; with other treatments later in the day

2. A patient with an infected wound has to have a bath before having his dressing done. Should you

   A. let him have his bath, then do his dressing before doing the other dressings
   B. let him have his bath while you are doing the other dressings, and then do his dressing last
   C. do the other dressings first, and let him have his bath and do his dressing afterwards

3. You are laying up a dressing trolley, and have a pre-sterilized pack containing the dressings and instruments. After cleaning the trolley, should you place the pack

   A. on the top shelf of the trolley
   B. on the bottom shelf

4. You have taken the trolley to a patient's bedside, drawn the curtains and put him in a suitable position. Should you next

   A. wash your hands, return to the bedside, then loosen the adhesive tape securing the dressing
   B. loosen the adhesive tape first, then wash your hands and return to the bedside

5. Which of the following is the correct method of washing hands before doing a dressing

    A. wash hands and dry them on a paper towel by the wash-bowl
    B. wash hands and leave them wet while you do the dressing
    C. wash hands and dry them on a sterile towel from the dressing pack

6. Which of the following is the correct method of dealing with soiled dressings

    A. discard all dressings into a paper bag which is emptied at the end of the dressing round into a special container (paper sack or bin) in the clinical room
    B. discard them into a paper bag which is emptied at the end of the dressing round into a special container in the sluice
    C. discard the paper bag after doing each dressing into a special container in the clinical room
    D. discard the paper bag after doing each dressing into a special container in the sluice

Now WRITE answers to the following questions.

7. In a few words show the stages by which bacteria may travel to a patient's wound

    (a) from a nurse with a sore throat or cold;
    (b) from a nurse with a boil.

Now correct your answers from the notes on pages 29 and 30.

ANSWERS AND NOTES ON REVISION QUIZ

For questions 1–6 count TWO marks for each correct answer.

Correct answer

1. B. One of the chief ways in which bacteria are carried to wounds is in *dust* in the air. Therefore dressings should be done as long as possible after bedmaking and cleaning. If cleaning, bedmaking or bed baths are going on, dust is being stirred up into the air, and can settle on trolleys or on the wound itself.

2. C. The infected patient's bath *and* dressing should be left until clean dressings have been done. Other patients may have to use the bath, so he should use it last; his wound should not be uncovered until all clean ones have been dressed.

3. B. The dressing pack should be on the bottom of the trolley. Its outer wrappings are not sterile, and may have picked up some dust. The top of the trolley is kept as clean as possible, for laying out dressings and instruments on sterile towels.

4. B. Loosen adhesive tape before washing hands. Once you have washed them, you handle everything with forceps.

5. A. Hands should be dried immediately on paper towel by the wash-bowl. Bacteria can stick more easily on anything wet. *Wet* hands can drip on the trolley or the wound, carrying bacteria on to them.

6. D. The soiled dressings from *each* wound must be discarded immediately. The paper bag containing them must be closed and put into a special sack or bin in the *sluice*. If taken back to the clinical room they may contaminate clean trolleys, etc.

For question 7 count marks as indicated.

7. (a) The various stages by which bacteria from the throat can reach a patient's wound are shown in the following diagram:

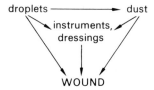

Count ONE mark for each of the above words mentioned = 5 marks.

(b) The stages are shown in the following diagram:

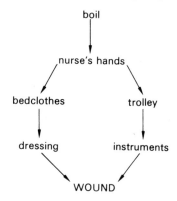

Count ONE mark for each of the above words mentioned = 7 marks.

Maximum Total = 24 marks.

Your score will show you how well you have done. Do any more revision which you think you need BEFORE attempting the question on the page opposite.

30

QUESTION

Without looking back or consulting any book, write the answer to the question
on this page. You should not take more than 40 minutes to plan and write your
answer.

You are nursing a patient who has an infected wound following an abdominal
operation.

(a) How could this wound have come infected?

(b) How would you prevent this infection from spreading to other parts of
the ward?

*When you have finished your answer, and not before, turn over and correct it
by the 'model answer' overleaf.*

MODEL ANSWER

(a) *Sources of infection* (50 marks)

The wound might have become infected by *dust* (4). Bacteria get into dust from droplets from noses and throats (2), which dry up on beds or floor (1). They can also get into dust from bedclothes (2), which can become contaminated with discharge from a wound (1) or discharging ear (1); or from soiled dressings dropped on bed or floor (2), or a split drainage bottle (1). Dust gets into the air (2), especially during bedmaking (2) or ward cleaning (2). It can settle on a wound while it is being dressed (2), or on instruments or dressings being used (2). It can also settle on bedclothes and so contaminate a wound (2).

Droplets from a nurse dressing the wound might have fallen on it (2). This would be specially dangerous if she had a sore throat (2).

Bacteria might have reached the wound by *indirect contact* (2). If a nurse had touched soiled dressing or instruments with her fingers (2), or had a boil or septic finger (1), she could carry them to the patient's bedclothes (1) or to instruments or dressings (2). She could infect the wound if she did not wash and dry her hands correctly before dressing it (2) or did not use non-touch technique (2). If soiled dressings had touched the trolley they could contaminate dressings or instruments (2).

The wound might have become infected from a *bath* if this had not been properly disinfected (3).

Possibly *instruments* or *dressings* were not properly sterilized (2), and so carried bacteria from another patient's wound (1).

(b) *Prevention of spread* (50 marks)

To prevent the infection from spreading, the infected wound should not be dressed until all clean ones have been done (4). The patient should not have a bath until after the patients with clean wounds (4), and afterwards the bath should be thoroughly cleaned and disinfected (3). His wound should be kept covered so that it does not discharge on to bedclothes (3), and he should be told not to touch his dressing (1). All nurses should wash their hands after making his bed or doing anything for him (3). If it was a very dangerous type of infection, the patient might be isolated in a side ward or sent to an isolation unit (2).

No dressings should be done while bedmaking is going on (2) or while the ward is being cleaned (2), or for an hour afterwards (2), so that there is as little dust in the air as possible (3).

Correct aseptic technique should be carried out in doing all the dressings (3); everything should be handled with forceps (3). Hands should be washed and dried on paper towels before each dressing (3).

Soiled dressings should be placed in paper bags without touching anything else (3), and instruments put into disinfectant (*or* paper bags) (3). Soiled things should not be taken into the clinical room where clean apparatus is kept (3); but put straight into the correct disposal sacks (*or* bins) in the sluice (3).

Surgical Nursing

6 CARE OF THE PATIENT WITH AN OVERACTIVE THYROID GLAND

REVISION QUIZ

In each of the following questions there is only ONE correct answer. You have to choose this; so write A, B or C, etc., ONLY.

1. Does the thyroid gland lie

    A. in front of the trachea   B. behind the trachea
    C. in the pharynx   D. in the thorax

2. Is thyroxine, which the thyroid produces

    A. a digestive juice   B. an enzyme
    C. a hormone

3. Does increased thyroxine

    A. increase the amount of calcium in the blood
    B. decrease the amount of calcium in the blood
    C. speed up the rate at which the body burns up food
    D. slow up the rate at which the body burns up food

4. Does a patient with thyrotoxicosis have

    A. a rapid pulse   B. a slow pulse

5. Does she

    A. gain weight   B. lose weight

6. Does she feel more comfortable

    A. in the summer   B. in winter

7. Is the patient's mental state

    A. confused   B. lethargic   C. excitable

8. Are her stools likely to be

    A. constipated   B. loose

9. Which of the following might be injured during an operation on the thyroid gland

    A. the trachea   B. the oesophagus
    C. the jugular vein   D. the nerves to the larynx

10. A patient has just returned from theatre after thyroidectomy. When she recovers consciousness, how would you nurse her

    A. in the semi-prone position
    B. lying flat with one pillow
    C. propped up with pillows

11. If her breathing appeared to be becoming distressed, would you

    A. give her oxygen
    B. give her a bed-table to lean over and extra pillows
    C. report it to the nurse in charge or the doctor

12. This patient finds swallowing difficult. Which of the following would you offer her

    A. water only   B. fruit juice with glucose
    C. egg custard

13. She also will not speak because her throat is sore. Which of the following would be the best way to help her

    A. give her a writing pad and pencil
    B. leave her alone until she feels better
    C. give her an aspirin gargle
    D. allow her fluids only

Now correct your answers from the notes on pages 37 and 38.

ANSWERS AND NOTES ON REVISION QUIZ

Count ONE mark for each correct answer.

Correct answer

1. A. In case you need reminding, the thyroid gland looks like this:

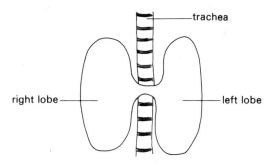

2. C. Digestive juices and enzymes are only found in the gastrointestinal
        tract. Hormones are produced by endocrine glands—the thyroid is
        one of these.

3. C. When the thyroid is over-active, metabolism (the rate at which the
        body burns its food) is speeded up. This accounts for the symptoms
        in questions 4–8 below.

4. A.

5. B.

6. A.

7. C.

8. B.

9. D. This is why one must observe whether or not the patient *can* speak after this operation. She will not *want* to speak as her throat is likely to be sore: the nurse must make sure which is the cause.

10. C. She will find it easier to breathe sitting up; her head and neck must be well supported. Drainage from her wound is helped.

11. C. This must be done at once. It may be due to blood collecting under the wound and causing pressure on her air passages.

12. C. Semi-solids are much easier to swallow.

13. C. This is best given before meals so eating will be easier also.

Maximum Total = 13 marks.

Your score will show you how well you have done. Do any more revision which you think you need BEFORE attempting the question on the page opposite.

QUESTION

Without looking back or consulting any book, write the answer to the question on this page. You should not take more than 40 minutes to plan and write your answer.

A 40-year-old patient in the ward is diagnosed as having an over-active thyroid gland.

(a) Where is the thyroid gland situated and what are the functions?

(b) List the specific observations you would make and report about this patient.

(c) If surgery is recommended, what immediate postoperative care will be required?

When you have finished your answer, and not before, turn over and correct it by the 'model answer' overleaf.

MODEL ANSWER

(a) *Position and functions* (15 marks)

The thyroid gland lies in front of the neck (3), over the trachea (2). It makes a hormone (2) called thyroxine (2) which is passed into the blood (1). This controls growth in infancy (1) and controls the rate of metabolism (*or* the rate at which the body converts food into energy) (4).

(b) *Observations* (25 marks)

Pulse: will be rapid (2). If it continues to increase (1) or becomes irregular (1) it must be reported at once as it may indicate heart failure (2). A sleeping pulse chart may be recorded half-hourly during the night and any changes reported (2).

Weight: the patient should be weighed daily as weight loss is often severe (2).

Appetite: this is usually very large (2) and the patient may be noticed eating between meals (1).

Emotional state: the patient may be very excitable and easily upset (2). The nurse should report if this happens or if the patient gets into an argument with another patient or member of staff (1).

Temperature: may be raised (1). She may complain of feeling hot and sweat a lot especially at night (2).

Sleep: often has insomnia (2). This should be reported as some sedation may be needed (1).

Periods: may stop (1) or be very heavy (1). This also must be reported by the nurse.

Bowels: she may complain of diarrhoea (1).

(c) *Immediate postoperative care* (60 marks)

On return, the patient is lifted onto a prepared bed (2) with one nurse supporting her head and neck (3). She is placed on her side to help maintain a good airway (2), with the head supported to prevent extension of the neck (1).

A waterproof sheet and towel are placed under her head and neck in case there is bleeding from the wound and a constant watch should be kept for this by the nurse who stays with the patient (4).

Pulse recordings are made at 15—30-minute intervals and any rise reported at once (4). The blood pressure may also be recorded if ordered (1).

When conscious the patient is sat upright with her head well supported (3). She can be washed and changed into her own nightgown, her hair combed and a mouthwash given (3). She should be given analgesics as prescribed as soon as necessary (3).

The amount of drainage should be reported as usually thyroidectomies have Redivac or similar drains inserted at operation (2).

Breathing must be checked frequently and any signs of distress reported at once as this may be caused by internal bleeding causing pressure on the air passages (4).

The patient should be kept fairly cool (1).

She may complain of a sore throat (2) or be afraid to speak (1) or swallow fluids (1), and will need constant reassurance that these symptoms will soon pass (1). Aspirin gargles or analgesic lozenges may be ordered before meals for a few days (2). The patient may find it easier to swallow thickened fluids and semi-solids (4) (*or* you may have given examples such as ice-cream, eggs, jellies, soup, mince, steamed fish, so count 1 mark for each up to 4 marks).

Hoarseness (1) and cramp or pains in the hands or feet (1) should be reported.

The nurse should encourage deep breathing exercises to prevent chest infection although it will be painful for the patient to cough (4). Mild analgesics may be prescribed to make it less uncomfortable for her (2).

The patient should also exercise her legs to prevent deep vein thrombosis (4) and will probably be allowed up the day after her operation when she will need help with walking at first (2). Care should be taken that the drainage bottle (*or* bottles) are supported (2).

Surgical Nursing

7 CARE OF VARIOUS DRAINAGE TUBES

REVISION QUIZ

In each of questions 1–6, there is only ONE correct answer. You have to choose this; so write A, B or C, etc., ONLY.

1. A patient has an indwelling catheter. You are asked to change his uribag. Should you

   A. wash your hands before you change the bag
   B. wash your hands after changing the bag
   C. wash your hands before and after changing it

2. For a patient with an indwelling catheter, would you

   A. restrict his fluid intake
   B. make sure he drinks 500 ml in 24 hours
   C. make sure he drinks 1000 ml in 24 hours
   D. let him drink as he wishes
   E. make sure he drinks 1500 ml in 24 hours
   F. make sure he drinks 5000 ml in 24 hours

3. A patient has a suction drain in his wound. When changing the bottle, should you

   A. allow the tube to drain into a receiver
   B. clamp the tube with artery forceps
   C. change the bottle quickly to prevent leakage

4. The surgeon would ask for a drainage tube to be removed from a wound when

   A. there was no further drainage
   B. after 48 hours
   C. if drainage were excessive
   D. after 10 days

5. When passing a nasogastric tube, would you know it is in the stomach when

      A. the tube has disappeared to mark '1' on the tube
      B. the patient coughs
      C. the tube disappears to mark '2'
      D. you aspirate material which turns blue litmus paper red
      E. the patient complains of nausea
      F. you aspirate material which turns red litmus paper blue

6. When passing a nasogastric tube, would you ask the patient to *swallow* when

      A. you insert the tube into his nostril
      B. he feels the tube at the back of his nose
      C. he feels the tube in his throat
      D. he starts to cough

7. What are the early signs of a urinary infection? There are FOUR correct answers. Pick them out from the list below:

A. rise of temperature	B. retention of urine
C. anuria	D. distension of bladder
E. low blood pressure	F. a rigor
G. subnormal temperature	H. high blood pressure
I. pain on passing urine	J. offensive urine

Now correct your answers from the notes on pages 45 and 46.

ANSWERS AND NOTES ON REVISION QUIZ

Count TWO marks for each correct answer.

Correct answer

1. C. It is important to wash your hands before you change a uribag because infection can easily travel upwards along the tubing and catheter into the bladder. It is obvious that you also wash *after* dealing with excreta of any kind, before you go on to another nursing task.

2. E. An adequate fluid intake helps to prevent urinary infection which is more likely to occur in a patient with an indwelling catheter. Fluids help to keep urinary output good and prevent it remaining in the bladder. Answer D. is too vague—he may just want to sleep and not bother to drink. Answer F. is improbable, to say the least.

3. B. This will prevent air entering the tube and making suction less effective. It also lessens the risk of bacteria entering the wound by means of the tube.

4. A. The whole purpose of a drain (of any kind) is to allow fluid to escape and not collect, stagnate and cause infection. The amount of drainage depends on where the tube is, and the type of operation. Some can be removed after 48 hours *if* there is no further drainage.

5. D. This indicates that you aspirate *acid* material and gastric juice *is* acid. Answers A. and C. are unreliable as patients differ in size and their oesophaguses also differ in length.

6. C. It helps the patient to tell him this before you start as it is impossible for him to keep swallowing and there is no point in making him over-anxious. It is too late when he starts to cough!

7. A. These all may be found when a urinary infection is beginning.
   F. They are thus important signs and symptoms which should
   I. be reported, especially if the patient has a catheter in
   J. place.

Maximum Total = 20 marks.

Your score will show you how well you have done. Do any more revision which you think you need BEFORE attempting the question on the opposite page.

QUESTION

Without looking back or consulting any book, write the answer to the question on this page. You should not take more than 40 minutes to plan and write your answer.

Describe what special observations and care are needed when a patient has each of the following tubes in position:

   (a) an indwelling catheter
   (b) a suction drain from a wound
   (c) a nasogastric tube

State the purpose of each tube.

When you have finished your answer, and not before, turn over and correct it by the 'model answer' overleaf.

MODEL ANSWER

(a) *Indwelling catheter* (34 marks)

Used to enable urine to drain from the bladder to relieve acute retention of urine or retention with overflow (4). Sometimes used to prevent pressure sores resulting from incontinence in unconscious or paralysed patients (2).

The patient must be encouraged to drink at least 2 litres of fluid each day (2); a fluid balance chart should be accurately recorded (2).

The nurse must make sure the catheter is draining freely (1) and that the tubing is not kinked, especially if the patient is up (2). The catheter usually drains into a uribag or other closed drainage system (1 for EITHER).

When the bag or bottle is changed, or emptied, care must be taken to avoid infection (1). The nurse must wash and dry her hands (2) and clamp off the tube before taking it from the bag (1). It is replaced by a sterile bag or bottle (2) (*or* count 5 marks for saying: after washing and drying the hands, certain types of uribag have the outlet released, the urine emptied into a measure jug, and the bag resealed).

The urethral orifice should be swabbed with cetrimide (*or* another example of antiseptic) to keep it free of secretions (2). This is done once or twice each day (1).

The catheter should be changed weekly will full aseptic precautions (2). The patient must not be allowed to touch the catheter (2). Bedclothes must be kept clean and dry (1). While the patient is up, the uribag must be supported by attaching it to his clothing (1).

Any signs of urinary infection should be reported at once: a raised temperature or pulse (1); a rigor (1) or an offensive (*or* 'fishy') smell from the urine (1). Specimens are sent regularly to the laboratory for testing (*or* bacterial examination) (2).

(b) *Suction drain from a wound* (33 marks)

This is usually used after mastectomy, cholecystectomy, amputations, thyroidectomy (4 for any TWO) or to prevent fluid forming between the pleura after chest surgery (3).

The bottle should be observed to make sure drainage is being maintained (3) as the reason for this tube is to prevent collections of blood (*or* haematomata) forming (2).

The type of drainage should be reported upon, especially if it alters (*or* if it becomes more blood-stained, cloudy or bile-stained) (3). When the bottle is changed, the amount of drainage should be charted as 'output' on the fluid balance chart (3).

When changing the bottle, the tube should be clamped to prevent air entering (*or* to maintain suction) (2). The new bottle must be sterile (2).

The wound area around the tube should not be touched and fresh sterile dressings only applied if necessary (3) using non-touch technique (*or* aseptic technique) (2). The patient should be asked not to touch the apparatus or the wound (2).

When the patient is up, the bottle should be supported or placed in a pocket (1) to prevent it from causing discomfort or from pulling out (3).

(c) *Nasogastric tube* (33 marks)

Used to aspirate the stomach contents (2) before and after surgery (2) on the stomach (1) and other parts of the alimentary tract (1). Used to prevent further vomiting in intestinal obstruction (2) and for giving stomach washouts in babies with pyloric stenosis (2). Used for feeding unconscious patients (2).

When the tube is in position for more than 24 hours, the nostril should be gently cleaned with bicarbonate of soda solution using small swabs wrapped round an orange-stick (3). Petroleum jelly can be applied around the edges of the nostril to keep the skin soft (2).

The tube is aspirated as often as instructed (2) and the aspirate observed for changes in appearance or content (2); these are reported (1) and the amounts measured and charted (2).

Between aspirations the tube is spigotted (1) and secured to the side of the patient's face with adhesive tape (1).

If it is used for feeding purposes, the tube is aspirated first and the aspirated tested with litmus paper (2), an acid reaction shows that the tube is in the stomach (2). Before and after the feed, 15−30 ml of water should be put down (2). The feed should always be allowed to pass down by gravity (1).

Surgical Nursing

8 OBSTRUCTIVE JAUNDICE

REVISION QUIZ

In questions 1–6 there is only ONE correct answer. You have to choose this;
so write, A, B or C, etc., ONLY.

1. Is an X-ray of the gall-bladder called

    A. a cholecystectomy   B. a barium meal
    C. a cholecystogram   D. an intravenous pyelogram
    E. a barium enema

2. Which of the following substances may appear in the urine when a
    patient is jaundiced

    A. blood   B. albumen   C. bile
    D. sugar   E. ketones

3. Which of the following organs is nearest to the gall-bladder

    A. the left lung   B. the right lung
    C. the heart   D. the oesophagus

4. Does the gall-bladder

    A. make bile   B. store bile

5. Are the contents of the gall-bladder discharged into the

    A. stomach   B. liver
    C. duodenum   D. jejunum

6. Is the patient who has gall-stones most often

    A. young and thin   B. short and fat
    C. middle-aged and thin   D. middle-aged and fat
    E. young and fat   F. tall and thin

Now WRITE answers to the following questions.

7. A patient returns from the theatre with a T-tube in position, having had his gall-bladder removed

    A. What drains from this tube?
    B. Where is the tube inserted?
    C. About how long is the tube left in?
    D. What is usually done before the tube is removed?

8. The patient also has a 'stab drain' (or Sterivac drain)

    A. What drains from this tube?
    B. Where is this tube inserted?
    C. About how long is this tube left in?

9. What would you report about

    (a) the T-tube
    (b) the stab drain

10. List the commonest complications and discomforts which may occur after this operation.

Now correct your answers from the notes on pages 53 and 54.

ANSWERS AND NOTES ON REVISION QUIZ

For questions 1–6 count TWO marks for each correct answer.

Correct answer

1. C. chole-=gall; -cysto=bladder; -gram=X-ray.

2. C. If there is obstruction to the bile passages, bile cannot escape and pigments become reabsorbed into the blood stream and are excreted in urine.

3. B. This is why a chest X-ray is usually taken prior to operation on the gall-bladder and also why the patient should be taught how to do breathing exercises. It also explains why chest complications are a particular hazard.

4. B. Bile is *made* in the liver, stored and excreted by the gall-bladder.

5. C. The diagram below will help to explain this if you have the answer wrong:

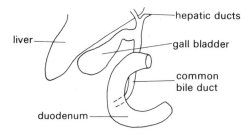

6. D. Some people best remember this by 'fair, fat and forty' ('fair' meaning the fair sex—women—rather than men).

For questions 7–10 count marks as indicated.

7. A. Bile (1).
    B. Into the common bile duct (2).
    C. 8–10 days (2).
    D. A special X-ray (choledochogram) of the bile ducts to find out whether bile can drain along them normally (3).

8. A. Blood-stained fluid (2).
    B. Into the gall-bladder bed (*or* the space left after the gall-bladder has been removed) (2).
    C. 2–3 days (*or* until it stops draining) (2).

9. (a) the amount of drainage each 24 hours (2)
         if the amount becomes suddenly increased (2)
         if it stops draining (2)
         when the tube is clamped off, if the patient complains of nausea (2)
    (b) if bile drains from it (4)
         if bleeding is excessive (2)
         if it stops draining (2)

10. Pain; 'wind' (*or* flatulence); nausea or vomiting; tightness of the chest or a cough (*or* inability to bring up sputum); constipation; deep-vein thrombosis; dislike of fatty foods.

     Count TWO marks for each you have mentioned.

     Possible total = 14 marks.

Maximum Total = 56 marks.

Your score will show you how well you have done. Do any more revision which you think you need BEFORE attempting the question on the page opposite.

QUESTION

Without looking back or consulting any book, write the answer to the question on this page. You should not take more than 40 minutes to plan and write your answer.

A middle-aged patient has gall-stones and is jaundiced.

   (a) What investigations may be carried out before surgery is considered?
   (b) Describe the special nursing care which will be required by this patient following operation.

When you have finished your answer, and not before, turn over and correct it by the 'model answer' overleaf.

MODEL ANSWER

(a) *Investigations* (20 marks)

Cholecystogram: the patient is given a dye which shows up the gall-bladder if it is functioning normally. The passage of the dye can be traced into the duodenum along the bile ducts (10). (If you have just said 'cholecystogram' count 4 marks.)

Urine testing: especially for bile (4).

Haemoglobin estimation (1).

Blood grouping and cross-matching so blood is ready for the operation (2).

Chest X-ray (2).

Liver function tests (1).

(b) *Special postoperative nursing care* (80 marks)

(NOTE TO STUDENT: this question asks for *special* care—meaning care only required after this particular operation.)

The patient returns from theatre with a T-tube in her common bile duct connected to a uribag (*or* other closed drainage system) (10). This tube allows some bile to pass into the duodenum and the rest to flow into the bag. It prevents the duct closing as it heals (5). It also prevents bile leaking into the peritoneum which would cause peritonitis (3). The drainage is measured and charted daily and lessens as more passes through the duct (3).

After 7–10 days, the tube is clamped off for increasing periods and the patient observed for nausea (3). An X-ray (*or* choledochogram) is usually taken before the tube is removed (3).

A stab (*or* suction) drain is also usually put in near the wound (3). The area around this is redressed daily with full aseptic (*or* non-touch) technique (2), the nurse reporting on the amount of drainage or the presence of bile (3) or pus (1). This drain is usually taken out after 48 hours. Sutures are removed after 8–14 days (2).

The patient may be overweight and find difficulty moving about the bed (2) or practising breathing exercises or leg movements (2). She will also have considerable pain and discomfort in her abdomen and will need frequent analgesics for the first 2–3 days (5). She will need help when she coughs, to support her wound while she expectorates (3) as the incision is usually high (*or* near the diaphragm) (2).

After 24 hours she can be helped out of bed with a nurse supporting her, and she should be encouraged to walk about to prevent deep vein thrombosis (3). Mobilization should be increased daily (1).

An enema or suppositories can be given on the third day to encourage a bowel action and relieve flatulence (2). Any bile in her urine must be reported (1).

At first there may be a nasogastric tube in the stomach to prevent postoperative vomiting (2). This must be aspirated as necessary and removed when the doctor orders, usually after 24 hours (2).

An intravenous infusion will probably have been put up in theatre and this is continued according to instructions until the patient is able to take oral fluids (2).

A little light diet can often be started after 24—36 hours (3), but fats should be avoided at first (3) as they may not be well tolerated. They should be introduced gradually (2) during her stay in hospital (2).

A period of convalescence is usually arranged by the social worker (2).

The patient can be discharged as soon as her wounds have healed—usually about 2 weeks after operation (1). A follow-up appointment is given for her to be seen in the out-patients department (2).

Surgical Nursing

9 CARE OF PATIENT WITH COLOSTOMY

REVISION QUIZ

In each of questions 1–4 you must refer to the diagram below. Each of these questions has only ONE correct answer, so choose this before writing A, B or C, etc., ONLY.

Diagram of intestine showing sites where 'ostomies' may be performed

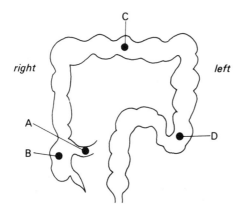

1. Would the patient's stools be the most liquid at site A, B, C or D?

2. Would the patient's stools be the most formed at site A, B, C or D?

3. D is commonly the site of a permanent colostomy, usually because the patient has

    A. intestinal obstruction   B. cancer of the rectum
    C. ulcerative colitis   D. obstruction in the caecum

4. If the opening were made at C, would the obstruction have been on the

    A. right of it   B. left of it   C. at 'C' itself

Now WRITE answers to the following questions.

5. Copy the diagram, labelling the parts of the intestine marked A to D.

6. List the requirements for redressing a colostomy.

7. List the different appliances you have seen used for patients with colostomies.

NOTE TO STUDENT. Useful reading on this subject may be found in:

How to Live with Your Colostomy (Abbott Laboratories Ltd) and *The Care of Your Colostomy* (London: Baillière Tindall).

Now correct your answers from the notes on pages 61 and 62.

ANSWERS AND NOTES ON REVISION QUIZ

For questions 1–4 count TWO marks for each correct answer.

Correct answer

1. A. This is the site for an *ileostomy* performed when the whole large intestine has to be removed. As one of the functions of the colon is to reabsorb water from the bowel's contents, this would not have occurred. Fluid stools are discharged from an ileostomy.

2. D. The faecal matter will have travelled almost the entire length of the colon and the stools will be almost normal in consistency, as the normal amount of water will have been absorbed.

3. B. When the rectum has to be removed, a permanent colostomy—also called a terminal colostomy—is performed at D. Not only are the stools formed, they can be regulated and the actual management of the stoma is easily learned by the patient. The site can also be reached easily for dressing purposes.

4. B. A colostomy is always performed *in front* of an obstruction.

For the questions 5—7 count marks as indicated.

5. A = ileostomy in *ileum* (*or* small bowel) (2)
    B = caecostomy in *caecum* (*or* ascending colon) (2)
    C = transverse colostomy in *transverse colon* (2)
    D = left iliac colostomy in *descending colon* (2)

6. Bowl of hot water (1); disposable washing-cloth, flannel or wool balls
    (1); soap or cetrimide in gallipot (1); towel (1); large disposal bag (1);
    fresh colostomy bag of same size and type as in use (1); scissors (1);
    adhesive tape or adhesive (1); gauze (1); cream or barrier cream (1);
    disposable gloves (1).

7. Only you know what you have seen used. If you have only seen one
    type, try to find out where you can see others: the School of Nursing will
    probably have one of each type in current use in your hospital. NO
    MARKS for this question.

Maximum Total = 27 marks.

Your score will show you how well you have done. Do any more revision
which you think you need BEFORE attempting the question on the page
opposite.

QUESTION

Without looking back or consulting any book, write the answer to the question on this page. You should not take more than 40 minutes to plan and write your answer.

A patient is to have an operation for a colostomy.

    (a) What is a colostomy?
    (b) What observations would you make during the first 24 hours after the operation?
    (c) Describe in detail how you would clean a colostomy after an evacuation.

When you have finished your answer, and not before, turn over and correct it by the 'model answer' overleaf.

MODEL ANSWER

(a) *What is a colostomy?* (15 marks)

A colostomy is an artificial opening from the colon (*or* large bowel) to the outside of the abdomen (6) through which faeces pass (3). It may be performed to relieve intestinal obstruction (3) or as a permanent measure when the rectum has to be removed (3).

(b) *Observations* (45 marks)

On return from the theatre, the patient's airway must be observed and suction used as necessary to keep it clear (3). As soon as he is conscious he should be encouraged to cough and expectorate and the nurse should report any breathing difficulties (3).

His pulse and blood pressure should be recorded half-hourly at first and any rise in pulse or fall in blood pressure reported at once (4). These observations can be less frequent as the patient's condition improves (2).

If the patient becomes pale (2) or cold and clammy (2), help should be summoned at once (2).

His temperature should be recorded four-hourly and any rise reported as this denotes infection (2).

Pain should be dealt with at once by giving the prescribed drugs (4) and nurse should note whether or not the pain was relieved (1).

A fluid balance chart is maintained (3) as the patient will probably be fed intravenously at first until the surgeon orders oral fluids (3). Urine output should be measured and it should be reported if no urine has been passed after 12 hours postoperatively (2).

Aspirations are also measured and charted from the nasogastric tube (2) and the type of aspirate noted (1).

The patient's wound (*or* wounds) should be inspected frequently and repacked as required (5). If there is much bleeding through the dressing it should be reported (1). The colostomy will probably need no attention during this time, but in some cases there may be drainage (*or* you may have said 'if there has been obstruction', there will be drainage from the colostomy) and this will need frequent attention (3).

(c) *Cleaning a colostomy* (40 marks)

Before starting a trolley or large tray should be set containing the following articles:

    a bowl of hot water
    disposable cloth, flannel or wool balls
    soap or cetrimide solution in gallipot

a large disposal bag
disposable gloves
towel
a fresh colostomy bag
adhesive tape or adhesive for the bag
scissors
gauze
cream for the skin
paper tissues

Count ONE mark for each item = 12 marks.

The patient may be worried about his colostomy at first and find any attention to it very distasteful. The nurse can help by trying to understand his feelings and by never showing her own anxieties or distaste when doing his dressing (2). She should gradually instruct him how to do it for himself and allow him to help as soon as he is well enough (2).

Privacy should be given by carefully drawing the bed-curtains and closing nearby windows (1). Later, the dressings can be done in the bathroom (1).

If there is also an operation wound, contamination by faeces should be avoided; it should be dressed separately using aseptic technique (2).

The nurse should wear disposable gloves (1). The used colostomy bag is removed, sealed and put in the disposal bag (2). Faecal matter should be gently cleaned away with paper tissues which are placed straight into the bag (2). The whole area is then washed with soap and water (1) and dried carefully (1). If the skin is sore, barrier cream may be used (2). Any rashes must be reported as some patients react to the adhesive or strapping and special treatment may be needed (2). The new bag is taken from its wrapper, the opening enlarged with scissors as necessary (1), so that it fits closely round the stoma (1). It is fixed in position with adhesive or strapping (1).

The nurse leaves the patient comfortable (2), clears away the equipment (1) and washes her hands (1) after discarding her gloves (1).

If the patient has helped, he also should wash his hands (1).

Surgical Nursing

10 OPEN FRACTURE OF THE TIBIA

REVISION QUIZ

In each of questions 1–7 there is only ONE correct answer. You have to choose this; so write A, B or C, etc., ONLY.

1. Which of the three bones in this diagram is the tibia?

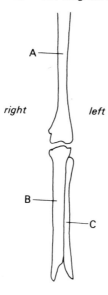

2. Is an open (or compound) fracture

    A. a fracture in which the bone is broken in several places
    B. one in which air can reach the broken bone
    C. one in which there is damage to internal organs
    D. one in which there is damage to nerves and blood vessels

3. When plaster of Paris is first applied in the treatment of a fractured tibia, will the plaster be

    A. padded   B. unpadded   C. hinged

4. Traction is often applied to a fracture of the tibia by means of a Steinman's pin. Is the pin inserted
    A. through the femur
    B. through the upper end of the tibia
    C. through the lower end of the tibia
    D. through the heel

5. Which of the following injuries is most likely to become infected with *anaerobic* bacteria
    A. a deep wound affecting muscles
    B. a burn
    C. a wound in which there is much loss of skin
    D. a cut with a knife

6. Which one of the following is caused by anaerobic bacteria
    A. a stitch abscess
    B. a carbuncle
    C. gas gangrene
    D. osteomyelitis (infection of bone)

7. Do anaerobic bacteria which cause disease commonly come from
    A. dust   B. air
    C. unwashed hands   D. earth

Now WRITE answers to the following questions.

8. A patient has just arrived in hospital with an open fracture of the tibia. List
    (a) the particulars you would take from him
    (b) any drugs which may be given before his fracture is treated in the operating theatre
    (c) the observations you would make before he went to theatre

9. Below is a list of things which may be done in the theatre. Put these *in order in which they would be done.*
    A. the fracture is reduced
    B. the wound is cleaned and dead tissue removed
    C. a Steinman's pin is inserted
    D. plaster of Paris is applied

10. List observations which should be made on the leg during the first few hours when the patient is in the ward.

Now correct your answers from the notes on pages 69–71.

ANSWERS AND NOTES ON REVISION QUIZ

For questions 1–7 count TWO marks for each correct answer.

Correct answer

1. B. The tibia is the larger of the two bones of the leg, on the inner side.

2. B. Open (or compound) fracture: one in which air can reach the broken bone through a wound. It therefore allows bacteria to enter.

3. A. The plaster is *padded* to allow room for swelling round the fracture. If it were not, the plaster would interfere with the blood supply of the leg.

4. D. A Steinman's pin is inserted through the bone of the heel (the os calcis or calcaneum). A stirrup is fastened to it, to which a cord with a weight can be attached, with the patient's leg in a Braun's frame. This prevents the two broken pieces of tibia from overlapping.

5. A. Anaerobic bacteria only multiply where there is no oxygen. Dead and damaged muscle is the best medium for them. Therefore an open fracture where the bone is surrounded by muscle, as with the tibia and femur, may be infected with this type of bacteria. Anaerobic bacteria particularly affect deep wounds.

6. C. Gas gangrene is caused by anaerobic bacteria, and is a very dangerous complication of an open fracture.
    Infection of the *bone* (osteomyelitis) is another danger; but is caused by aerobic, not anaerobic bacteria.

7. D. Tetanus and gas gangrene organisms, both anaerobic, are present in earth. As compound fractures are often caused by accidents in which there is contamination with soil, both these are dangers.

For questions 8–10 count marks as indicated.

8. (a) Full name and address; age, religion; name and address of next of kin; telephone number (1 mark for each = 5).
   (b) An analgesic (*or* drug to relieve pain) (1). Examples: morphine, omnopon, pethidine (1 for any example).
       An antibiotic to prevent infection by aerobic and anaerobic bacteria (1). Penicillin and ampicillin are effective against gas gangrene and tetanus organisms as well as against the usual aerobic ones.
       Tetanus toxoid is usually given also (1).
       Atropine will be given before the patient goes to the theatre (1) to prevent respiratory complications.
   (c) Temperature (1); pulse and respirations (1); blood pressure (1); urine testing (1).

9. The correct order is: B, A, C, D (2 marks).

   (a) The skin is shaved and cleaned and dead tissue cut out before the fracture is treated. It is sutured if possible; this makes the open fracture into a closed one.
   (b) The fracture is reduced. Reduction means manipulating the bone so that the pieces are in the correct position.

(c) If a Steinman's pin is to be used, it is inserted and then embedded in the plaster.

(d) Plaster of Paris is applied to immobilize the fracture.

10. Observe whether toes become cold (1) or blue (1). This would show that the circulation of blood was being interfered with. Observe whether patient can move toes (1). Observe any fresh bleeding through plaster (1); whether there is soreness round the edges of the plaster (1); and whether the patient is having much pain in the leg (1).

Maximum Total = 36 marks.

Your score will show you how well you have done. Do any more revision which you think you need BEFORE attempting the question on the page opposite.

QUESTION

Without looking back or consulting any book, write the answer to the question on this page. You should not take more than 40 minutes to plan and write your answer.

A young man is admitted with an open (or compound) fracture of the tibia following a motor cycle accident.

(a) What is meant by an open (or compound) fracture, and what are the special dangers of such an injury?

(b) Outline the admission procedure and the immediate treatment which this patient would receive on arrival in hospital.

(c) List the observations you would make on his leg during the first night after his admission.

When you have finished your answer, and not before, turn over and correct it by the 'model answer' overleaf.

MODEL ANSWER

(a) *Open fracture and its dangers* (15 marks)

An open (or compound) fracture is one in which the broken bone is exposed to the air (*or* in which there is a wound going down to the broken bone) (5).

Special dangers are infection of the bone through the wound (*or* osteomyelitis) (2) and infection by anaerobic organisms (*or* anaerobic bacteria) (2), causing gas gangrene (3) or tetanus (3).

(b) *Admission and immediate treatment* (70 marks)

Trousers are cut off the injured leg (2) and the patient is gently undressed (1) and examined by a doctor (1). He will be given an analgesic (*or* a drug to relieve pain) (3), such as pethidine, morphine or omnopon (1 for any example). He will also be given an antibiotic (3), such as penicillin or ampicillin (1 mark for any example), and tetanus toxoid (3). The leg may be temporarily immobilized with a splint to prevent pain (1) while an X-ray of his leg is taken (2).

His particulars are taken, including full name and address (1), age (1), religion (1), name and address of next of kin (1) and telephone number (1). His relatives are informed (2), if necessary by the police (2). He is asked to sign a form of consent to operation (3). The person taking his particulars finds out when he last had a meal (3).

His urine is tested (3). His temperature (1), pulse (1), respiration (1) and blood pressure (1) are taken (2) and charts made out (2). Before going to theatre he has an injection of atropine (2).

In theatre a general anaesthetic is given (2). The leg is cleaned and shaved (3); dead tissue is cut away (3) and the wound sutured (2). The fracture is then reduced (3). It will then be immobilized in plaster of Paris (3), which is padded to allow for swelling (2), or a Steinman's pin may be inserted through the heel (2) so that traction can be applied (2) with the leg in a Braun's frame (1).

(c) *Observations on the leg* (15 marks)

The nurse would observe whether the patient's toes became blue (3) and cold (3), and whether he could move them (2); whether there is any fresh bleeding through the plaster (3); whether the edges of the plaster cause soreness (2); whether the patient complains of pain in the leg (2).

Surgical Nursing

11 HEAD INJURY: CARE OF THE UNCONSCIOUS PATIENT

REVISION QUIZ

In each of questions 1–7 there is only ONE correct answer. You have to choose this; so write A, B or C, etc., ONLY.

1. In which of the following positions would you nurse a deeply unconscious patient

   A. on his back with head to one side
   B. on his side
   C. semi-prone
   D. propped up with several pillows

2. Would you take the pulse and blood pressure of an unconscious patient with a head injury

   A. twice a day   B. four-hourly
   C. two-hourly   D. half-hourly

3. If a patient is becoming more deeply unconscious, does the pulse rate

   A. become more rapid   B. become slower

4. If a patient is becoming more deeply unconscious, does the blood pressure

   A. rise   B. fall

5. You are testing the pupil reactions of a patient with a head injury. Do you shine your torch

   A. into either one of his eyes
   B. into each eye separately
   C. into both eyes at the same time

6. Which of the following would be a *normal* pupil reaction

    A. for both pupils to constrict (become smaller) equally
    B. for both pupils to dilate (become larger) equally
    C. for both pupils to remain the same size

7. Should the temperature of an unconscious patient be taken

    A. in the mouth   B. in the axilla   C. in the rectum

Now WRITE answers to the following questions.

8. Write short notes on the attention required to (a) the eyes; (b) the mouth; (c) the pressure areas; (d) the bowels and (e) the bladder of a deeply unconscious patient.

9. List the steps you would take in giving a feed through a nasogastric (Ryle's) tube to an unconscious patient.

Now correct your answers from the notes on pages 77 and 78.

ANSWERS AND NOTES ON REVISION QUIZ

For questions 1–7 count TWO marks for each correct answer.

Correct answer

1. C. In the semi-prone position the patient is less likely to asphyxiate. His jaw falls forward, so that his tongue cannot obstruct his air way; and saliva, secretions or blood trickle out instead of being inhaled.

2. D. Pulse and blood pressure are taken *frequently*, as changes can occur which show a change in the depth of consciousness.

3. B.⎫ *Fall* in pulse rate and *rise* in blood pressure occur when a
4. A.⎭ patient with a head injury is becoming more deeply unconscious.

5. B. Shine torch into each eye separately.

6. A. Pupils normally *constrict* (become smaller) when they react to light. Both should react briskly and equally.

7. C. Temperatures taken in the rectum are more accurate than those taken in the axilla. Obviously you cannot use the mouth in an unconscious patient.

For questions 8 and 9 count marks as indicated.

8. (a) Swab each eye separately with normal saline or cooled boiled water (1), instil drops or ointment if ordered (1), keep eyes closed, with strapping if necessary (1).
   (b) Secretions should first be removed by suction (1). Clean mouth with sodium bicarbonate solution, then glycerine of thymol or other mouthwash, then glycerine and lemon or glycerine to draw moisture into the mouth (3).
   (c) The patient must be *turned* each time he is attended to (1). Pressure areas are kept clean and dry (1).
   (d) It is important to report bowel actions and note if there are none (1). Suppositories may be needed (1).
   (e) A patient who is unconscious for any length of time will usually have Paul's tubing over the penis, or else a self-retaining catheter (1). See that drainage tubing is not kinked (1) measure and report output each time the uribag is emptied (1).

9. Aspirate the nasogastric tube (1) and record the amount as output (1). Attach the barrel of the syringe and pour in a small quantity of water to clear the tube (1). Pour in the feed (1) and record the amount on the fluid chart (1). Clear the tube with water (1).

Maximum Total = 34 marks.

Your score will show you how well you have done. Do any more revision which you think you need BEFORE attempting the question on the page opposite.

QUESTION

Without looking back or consulting any book, write the answer to the question on this page. You should not take more than 40 minutes to plan and write your answer.

A patient is admitted to your ward following a head injury. He is unconscious.

(a) What position will you nurse him in and why?
(b) What observations will you make and record?
(c) Describe the nursing care he will require.

When you have finished your answer, and not before, turn over and correct it by the 'model answer'. overleaf.

MODEL ANSWER

(a) *Position* (15 marks)

This should be semi-prone (5) with no pillow (1). This allows the jaw and tongue to fall forward (2) and any secretions to run out of the patient's mouth (2); and therefore lessens the danger of asphyxia (5).

(b) *Observations* (35 marks)

Observations are made and recorded hourly or half-hourly (3) on the pulse rate and respirations (3) and blood pressure (3), and on the reaction of the pupils to light (3). It should be recorded whether pupils constrict equally when a torch is shone into each separately (1), or whether one or both does not constrict (1). At the same time the nurse records whether the patient appears to react to any stimulus (1), e.g. when he is touched or moved (2), or whether he takes any notice when she speaks to him (2), or reacts to pain (1).

All fluid being given by nasogastric (*or* Ryle's tube) or intravenously is recorded (2), and the output of urine from an indwelling catheter or Paul's tubing on the penis (2). If he has a nasogastric tube aspirations from it are also recorded (2).

The temperature is taken rectally (2) every four hours (1), or hourly at first (1).

The urine is tested regularly for abnormalities (2), and the results recorded each time (1). Bowel actions must also be recorded (2).

(c) *Nursing care* (50 marks)

The patient needs attention about every two hours (4).

Secretions are removed from the mouth and nose with a suction apparatus (2), using separate sterile catheters for each (1). The mouth is cleaned (3) with sodium bicarbonate (1), glycerine of thymol (*or* other mouthwash) (1), and glycerine and lemon (1), and cold cream is applied to the lips (1).

The eyes are swabbed with normal saline (3), any drops or ointment ordered are instilled (2) and the lids are closed (2). Lids may have to be kept closed with strips of strapping (2).

The patient is turned regularly (*or* two-hourly) on to his other side (3), and his pressure areas are washed, dried and powdered (3). Passive movements are done to exercise all his joints (3).

If urine is draining into a uribag, this is emptied (2). If the patient is being fed through a nasogastric (*or* Ryle's) tube, this is aspirated (3). About 30 ml of water are put down using the barrel of a syringe (2) to clear the tube (1). His

80

two-hourly feed, such as Complan, is then poured down (3), and the tube again cleared with water (1).

The patient will need bed bathing each day (2), and attention given to his hair (1) and nails (1).

He may require suppositories if his bowels do not open (2).

Geriatric Nursing

12 TRANSFER AND DISCHARGE OF PATIENTS

1. Imagine that YOU are an elderly patient in an acute medical ward. You have been told that you have to go to another hospital, specially for elderly patients.

   (a) list the questions you would want to ask of the nurse
   (b) list the questions your relatives would want to ask

2. What special nursing care would this patient need? List her requirements

   (a) the day before her transfer
   (b) the day of her transfer

3. What will she need to take with her? List the items that should accompany this patient.

4. What steps will you take to help an elderly patient prepare herself for independence?

5. List the arrangements that need to be made before an elderly patient returns to her own home after a long stay in hospital.

Now correct your answer from the notes on pages 85 and 86.

ANSWERS AND NOTES ON REVISION QUIZ

Count marks as indicated.

1. (a) Why am I being sent away from here? (2)
       Where is the other hospital? (2)
       Will my relatives be told? (2)
       Will they be allowed to visit? (2)
       Will I have the same doctor to look after me? (1)
       Will I be there long? (2)
       Will I be allowed up? (1)
       (If 'you' have any special likes and dislikes, you would also worry
       about these and having to explain to new people) (THREE for any
       suggestion)
   (b) Why is she going? (2)
       When will she go? (1)
       Will we be allowed to visit? (1)
       How will we get there? (2)
       How will the patient get there? (1)
       Will she get the same attention there? (2)
       (You may have thought of other relevent points not mentioned
       here— discuss these with your colleagues and count marks if
       suitable.)

   Possible total = 24 marks.

2. (a) Bath (2)
       Wash hair (2)
       Attend to nails (2)
       Clean clothing for next day (2)
       Outdoor clothing if patient is to be dressed (2)
       Ask relatives to bring a suitcase or carrier (2)
       Find out who is to accompany the patient (2)
   (b) Bath (2)
       Help with dressing (2)
       Help with packing (2)
       Reassurance (2)
       Comfort while waiting (2)
       Tell her what time she will be fetched (2)

   Possible total = 26 marks.

3. All her belongings from her locker (*or* specify items) (3)
Any books, papers, letters, plants she has (2)
Case notes and X-rays (in some hospitals *only*) (2)
A note from the sister to the sister in the geriatric hospital (2).

Possible total = 9 marks.

4. Help her to wash (*or* bath) and dress herself (2). Let her help to make her own bed (1) and encourage her to look after her clothes and wash small items (1). Let her help to make tea and serve meals to the other patients (1). Suggest other tasks she can assist in: arranging flowers in ward, dusting, washing-up, etc. (1). Take her out in the garden for short periods (1) and encourage her visitors to take her on short trips (1).

You may be able to think of other ideas; discuss these with your colleagues and if they are thought suitable, count TWO marks each for up to FOUR further suggestions.

Possible total = 16 marks.

5. The hospital social worker (1) may contact the Social Services Department (1) of the Local Authority in the area where the patient lives and it is then the Department's responsibility to obtain equipment (1), arrange any adaptations to the home (1), and alert services such as Home Help and Meals-on-Wheels (1). In many cases the Department will liaise with the health visitor (*or* the geriatric visitor) (1) and the general practitioner (1) to ensure that the home is in a suitable state for the patient to return (1). These arrangements can not normally be made by the hospital nurse herself.

Possible total = 8 marks.

Maximum Total = 83 marks.

Your score will show you how well you have done. Do any more revision which you think you need BEFORE attempting the question on the page opposite.

QUESTION

Without looking back or consulting any book, write the answer to the question on this page. You should not take more than 40 minutes to plan and write your answer.

What preparations would you make for an elderly patient

(a) to be transferred from an acute ward to a geriatric hospital
(b) to be discharged home from the geriatric hospital

When you have finished your answer, and not before, turn over and correct it by the 'model answer' overleaf.

MODEL ANSWER

(a) *Transfer of patient from acute ward* (50 marks)

Adequate explanation must be given to the patient (2) and her relatives (2) as soon as possible (2). They should be told about the reasons for the patient's transfer (2) and the better facilities in the geriatric hospital are stressed (2).

The relatives may be elderly and need information about the visiting times, and how to reach the new hospital, and any other points which will be helpful and reassuring to them (3 for any 2 suggestions).

For the day of transfer, transport will have to be arranged (3) and a relative asked to accompany the patient if possible (3). If not, an escort (*or* a nurse, voluntary worker, Red Cross escort) should be detailed to go with the patient (2 for any 1 suggestion).

On the day of transfer, the patient is given a bath (3). Her hair should have been recently washed (2); finger- and toenails should be seen to be short and clean (2). If possible suitable day clothes are worn (3); if not, warm, clean nightclothes are put on covered with a dressing-gown (3). Legs and feet should be warm—preferably stockings and slippers worn as elderly people feel the cold (2). She should be left comfortably in a chair to await transport with a rug around her legs (2); she must be given drinks or meals while waiting (1).

A nurse should help the patient pack her belongings—or pack for her—in a suitcase or carrier-bag, which should be labelled with her name (4).

Sometimes case-notes and X-rays are sent with the patient and if so they should be up to date and put in a sealed envelope addressed to the sister at the geriatric hospital (3). The sister of the acute ward may also write a note about any nursing information which might be helpful (1).

A nurse should take the patient to the front door and hand her over to her escort, reassuring the patient that she will soon settle down in her new 'home' (3).

(b) *Discharge of patient home from geriatric hospital* (50 marks)

The nursing staff should talk to the patient about going home (3) so that any worries she may have can be discussed (1). She may have been in hospital some time and have become dependent; she should be encouraged to do more for herself so she gains self-confidence (3) such as dressing herself in day clothes, bathing herself, washing her stockings etc., making tea and preparing bread and butter, making her own bed (2 for any 2 suggestions of tasks she may do).

Relatives should also take part in the discussions about the care the patient will need at home (2); they will probably need reassurance that she will be able to manage and that she will be visited by her general practitioner (2). If she needs visits from the community nurse or health visitor, this will be arranged by her doctor (2).

The social worker may have made a home visit to find out if any alterations or aids need to be attended to (*or* you may have actually stated aids such as commode, bath rail, hand-rail on either side of lavatory, walking-frame, laundering service) (2 for any 2 suggestions). A Home Help may be needed (1).

Before discharge, the patient should be up and dressed for most of the day and it may be possible to allow her out in the grounds for short walks (2); her relatives may be able to take her out for a drive, or home to tea or for the weekend (2 for any suggestion).

Immediately prior to her discharge, the nurse should check with the social worker, if possible in front of the patient, that arrangements have been made for food to have been bought (3) and that her house will have been aired (*or* warmed) (3).

Some form of transport should be arranged (2); if possible a relative or neighbour should be asked to fetch her (2). Suitable outdoor clothes should be brought in for the journey (2).

A nurse should help the patient pack her belongings if she cannot do this by herself (3); the nurse makes sure she does not leave anything behind or take hospital property away in error (3). She is helped to dress (2) and should wait in a comfortable chair until fetched (3). Any valuables are fetched from the hospital safe and signed for by the patient (2).

A nurse should escort the patient to the front door and see that she is well wrapped up if the weather is cold (3).

Geriatric Nursing

13 HEMIPLEGIA

In each of questions 1—8 there is only ONE correct answer. You have to choose this; so write A, B or C, etc., ONLY.

1. Is hemiplegia

   A. paralysis of the lower half of the body
   B. paralysis of one side of the body

2. Is the usual cause of hemiplegia

   A. damage to the brain through a head injury
   B. damage to the spinal cord
   C. interference to the blood supply of the brain on the paralysed side
   D. interference to the blood supply on the opposite side of the brain

3. In a patient with hemiplegia, do the joints become

   A. stiff in a bent position
   B. limp and relaxed
   C. stiff and unable to bend
   D. limp and contracted

4. Does 'passive movement' of a patient's joints mean that

   A. she is encouraged to move her own limbs
   B. a physiotherapist or nurse moves them for her

5. Does 'active movement' mean that

   A. the patient moves her own limbs
   B. someone else moves them for her

6. If an elderly patient has hemiplegia, is it better

   A. to nurse her in bed until movement returns to her limbs
   B. to sit her out in a chair with her shoes on
   C. to sit her in a chair with her feet elevated

7. When giving this patient a meal, would you

    A. feed her before the food gets cold
    B. leave the food on her locker and say 'you can feed yourself'
    C. cut up her food and say 'try to feed yourself'

8. Do you consider that this patient's spectacles and false teeth should be

    A. kept in a safe place such as sister's office until she is better
    B. put in her locker where she can reach them
    C. put in her locker out of her reach so that a nurse can give them to her if necessary

Now WRITE answers to the following questions.

9. List all the joints which need exercising when a patient has hemiplegia.

10. A foot board and bed cradle can be put in the bed in order to prevent one of the complications of hemiplegia. Name this complication.

11. Apart from those directly caused by her paralysis, list two other difficulties which a patient with hemiplegia may have.

Now correct your answers from the notes on pages 93 and 94.

ANSWERS AND NOTES ON REVISION QUIZ

For questions 1–8 count TWO marks for each correct answer.

Correct answer

1. B. Paralysis of one side.

2. D. The muscles on each side of the body are controlled by nerve
       impulses coming from the *opposite* side of the brain, as shown in
       the diagram below.

          Hemiplegia is usually caused by a 'cerebrovascular accident', i.e.
       a thrombosis or haemorrhage of blood vessels on the opposite side
       of the brain.

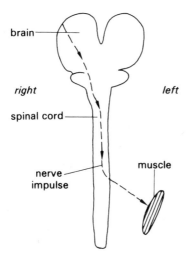

3. A. Joints become *spastic*, i.e. stiff, and they are in a position of flexion
       (bent). Unless rehabilitation is started quickly, hips and knees may
       become contracted so that walking is impossible. The fingers may
       also be bent so that the patient cannot use her hand.

4. B. 'Passive movements' are done for the patient.

5. A. 'Active movements' are those which she does for herself.

6. B. The aim is to help the patient to move as much as possible. Having her shoes on makes it easier for her to stand, and, later, to walk.

7. C. Trying to feed herself is part of the patient's rehabilitation; but she cannot do so unless she is in a convenient position and is helped if necessary.

8. B. You want the patient to become as independent as possible. She will feel very helpless and frustrated if she cannot get at her spectacles and false teeth. If you chose any other answer, you should read *Sans Everything* by B. Robb!

For questions 9–11 count marks as indicated.

9. Shoulder (1), elbow (1), wrist (1), fingers (1), thumb (1), hip (1), knee (1), ankle (1), toes (1).

10. Foot drop (1).

11. Incontinence (2); loss of speech (2).

Maximum Total = 30 marks.

Your score will show you how well you have done. Do any more revision which you think you need BEFORE attempting the question on the page opposite.

QUESTION

Without looking back or consulting any book, write the answer to the question on this page. You should not take more than 40 minutes to plan and write your answer.

What is hemiplegia?

What can the nurse do for a patient with this condition

    (a) to prevent deformities
    (b) to assist with his rehabilitation

When you have finished your answer, and not before, turn over and correct it by the 'model answer' overleaf.

MODEL ANSWER

Hemiplegia is paralysis of one side of the body (3), usually due to a cerebrovascular accident (*or* cerebral thrombosis *or* haemorrhage) (1) on the opposite side of the brain (1).

(a) *Prevention of deformities* (40 marks)

The paralysed limbs must be supported in as natural a position as possible (3). If the patient is unconscious or has to stay in bed, a foot board at the bottom of the bed is used to prevent foot-drop (3); if she is sitting out of bed, she should wear a shoe on the affected foot (2) and it should be flat on the floor (1). A paralysed arm can be supported on a pillow (2), and a roll of bandage or a ball should be put in the hand to prevent the finger joints becoming contracted (*or* permanently bent) (3). The hip (1) and knee joint (1) should be kept as straight (*or* extended) as possible (1), and a pillow between the legs is used to help this (2).

A bed cradle must be used to keep off the weight of the bedclothes (2) and to allow the patient to move while in bed if she can (2). The nurse should encourage her to move all her joints as soon as she can (2) and whenever she is attended to (1). The nurse should also do 'passive movements' on all the joints if the patient cannot move them herself (4), including the hip (1), knee (1), ankle (1), toes (1), shoulder (1), elbow (1), wrist (1), fingers (1) and thumb (1), especially at times when the physiotherapist cannot come (1).

(b) *Rehabilitation* (55 marks)

As soon as possible, the patient should be got up to sit in a chair (2), and encouraged to take a few steps as soon as she can (2), holding on to the bed (1) or with the help of nurses (1). This will be easier if she wears her own shoes (2).

She should be encouraged to use her good arm to help feed herself (2), wash (2) and dress herself (2), and helped to do her own hair (2). The nurse must give her sufficient help, or she will get discouraged (3). For example, she will need some of her food cut up (2), and she must be able to reach things with her good hand (2). The nurse must always be patient and encouraging (2).

The nurse must encourage her to do the exercises which the physiotherapist has taught her as often as possible (2); and when she is learning to walk again must be ready to help her (2).

She may be incontinent at first (3), so the nurse must see that she uses a commode or bedpan (2) about every two hours (2), and must not keep her waiting for attention (1).

It will help her if she is kept interested (3), and visitors should be welcomed (3). She is also encouraged to use her hands for knitting or weaving if she can (2), to read (1) and to take an interest in the ward (1). She must be allowed to wear her own clothes (2), and her spectacles and false teeth must be within her reach (3).

If she has lost her speech, the nurse can explain to visitors that she can still understand them, and encourage them to talk to her (3).

Geriatric Nursing

14 NEGLECT AND MALNUTRITION

REVISION QUIZ

For questions 1–8 there is only ONE correct answer. You have to choose this; so write A, B or C, etc., ONLY.

1. A 'good diet' is one which contains correct amounts of the essential food factors in each 24 hours. Which of the following is the best diet? One which contains

    A. 100 g carbohydrate, 400–500 g fat and 100 g protein
    B. 400–500 g carbohydrate, 100 g fat and 400–500 g protein
    C. 100 g carbohydrate, 100 g fat and 100 g protein
    D. 400–500 g carbohydrate, 100 g fat and 100 g protein
    E. 100 g carbohydrate, 100 g fat and 400–500 g protein
    F. 400–500 g carbohydrate, 400–500 g fat and 100 g protein

2. Which of the following groups contains only first-class protein?

    A. peas, beans, lentils, nuts, cheese
    B. fish, meat, cheese, eggs, milk
    C. milk, bread, tomatoes, cabbage, butter
    D. eggs, milk, oranges, nuts, raisins

3. Why is milk called the 'perfect food'? Is it because it

    A. is easily digested   D. contains a good amount of iron
    B. is best for babies   E. has all the food factors
    C. contains all the vitamins

4. Why is fat needed in the diet? Is it to

    A. prevent loss of body weight   B. maintain body temperature
    C. assist with growth   D. guard against colds

5. In the diet, is protein needed for

    A. guarding against colds   B. growth and repair
    C. healthy teeth and gums   D. maintaining body temperature

6. Are carbohydrates required for

    A. preventing infections   B. growth and repair
    C. preventing anaemia   D. providing heat and energy

7. Choose the line below in which *all* the foods contain vitamin C.

    A. milk, oranges, chocolate, bread
    B. meat, bananas, cabbage, strawberries
    C. oranges, new potatoes, fish, meat
    D. grapefruit, blackcurrants, salad, lemons

8. Is vitamin C needed to

    A. promote healing   B. help clotting
    C. make strong teeth   D. provide energy

Now WRITE answers to the following questions.

9. All the food we eat is metabolized (burnt by the body) and produces heat which is measured in *Calories*. From the list below, select the correct number of Calories required by

    (a) a manual worker
    (b) a student nurse
    (c) a secretary
    (d) an unconscious patient
    (e) an elderly lady confined to bed

    A. 4000   B. 3200   C. 3000
    D. 2000   E. 1500   F. 1000
    G. 500

10. A patient is admitted in a state of neglect. Fill in the chart below with *notes* on how neglect affects each.

Skin	Hair	Mouth	Bowels	Mental Outlook

Now correct your answers from the notes on pages 101 and 102.

ANSWERS AND NOTES ON REVISION QUIZ

For questions 1–8, count ONE mark for each correct answer.

Correct answer

1. D. Carbohydrates are the bulky foods which prevent hunger—we need most of these. Incidentally, these are the foods to cut down if we wish to lose weight.

2. B. These all contain 'first-class proteins'—expensive foods. Nuts, vegetables like peas, beans and lentils contain second-class proteins, less valuable to the body. Baked beans are popular and useful, cheap and hunger preventing (because of the carbohydrates in the sauce), but not as useful as the foods in B.

3. E. A and B are also *true*, but does not make milk the perfect food for everyone. It contains very little vitamin C and NO iron.

4. B. It yields a large amount of Calories.

5. B. This is because all body cells contain protein in the protoplasm.

6. D. The more heat and energy we require, the more carbohydrates we eat, dictated to by our appetites.

7. D. Oranges, lemons, grapefruit, blackcurrants are 'citrus' fruits and are the best sources of this vitamin. Many of the foods listed are only eaten when cooked, and cooking destroys vitamin C.

8. A. Helps in the manufacture of new cells.

9.   (a) = A   (b) = B or C   (c) = C
    (d) = D   (e) = D

    Count TWO marks for each correct answer.

10. Count marks as indicated:

Skin: dirty (1); offensive smell (1); sore where two surfaces rub (1); long, horny nails (1); areas of broken skin (1); skin infections (*or* boils, impetigo, septic spots) (1).

Hair: tangled (1); dirty (1); greasy (1); infested with nits or lice (1); impetigo (*or* septic spots) of scalp (1).

Mouth: decayed and broken teeth (1); offensive breath (*or* halitosis) (1); furred tongue (1); ulcerated mucous membrane (1); cracked lips (1); infected glands (*or* parotitis) (1).

Bowels: constipation (*or* impacted faeces) (1); diarrhoea if severely undernourished (1).

Mental outlook: lethargy (1); withdrawn (*or* uncommunicative) (1); uncooperative (*or* resentful of help) (1).

Maximum Total = 40 marks.

Your score will show you how well you have done. Do any more revision which you think you need BEFORE attempting the question on the page opposite.

QUESTION

Without looking back or consulting any book, write the answer to the question on this page. You should not take more than 40 minutes to plan and write your answer.

An elderly patient is admitted to your ward suffering from neglect and malnutrition.

(a) Describe the nursing care which this patient would require.
(b) What diet may be ordered?

When you have finished your answer, and not before, turn over and correct it by the 'model answer' overleaf.

MODEL ANSWER

(a) *Nursing care* (75 marks)

It is important that the nurses gain the patient's confidence as elderly people may find difficulty getting used to new routines, new people or a change in environment (3 for any 2 suggestions). The patient should be greeted by name (2) and two nurses should help lift her into bed (2).

The patient may be able to give her own personal particulars; if not, a relative, neighbour or friend may be asked to do so (3).

Her temperature, pulse and respirations are taken and recorded daily (1), but if these are abnormal (*or* higher or lower than normal) may be taken four-hourly (1).

The patient is given a bath, or bed bath, according to her condition (2). The nurse must report on the condition of her skin, especially any areas of broken skin, bruises or rashes (3). Nails should be carefully cleaned and cut (2). It may also be necessary to wash her hair (2) and signs of nits or lice should be reported on and dealt with at once (2).

If the patient has dentures, these should be removed and cleaned (2); her mouth should be examined to see if the mucous membrane is healthy (1) and the tongue moist or dry (1). Her teeth can then be replaced (1).

During these procedures, the patient should be kept as warm as possible (2) and the nurse should talk kindly to her to get to know her (2). Afterwards, she can be given a warm drink and allowed to rest quietly (3).

The patient should be given a bell and told how to summon a nurse (2).

When she uses a bed-pan, her urine should be tested and any abnormalities reported and charted (4).

The nurse should be able to report on the patient's general condition: whether she can see, hear, move her limbs and answer questions rationally (3 for any 3 points you have mentioned). She may also tell nurse about her relatives (1), whether she has anyone to look after her home (1) or whether she has any pets which need caring for (1). The social worker may be contacted to relieve the patient's anxiety about any of these problems (2).

As soon as her condition allows, the patient should be allowed up (2). If necessary, attractive, well-fitting clothes should be obtained for her (2) and she should be encouraged to mix with other patients (2).

Suitable diversional or occupational therapy will help to restore the patient's morale and sense of independence (3); friends can be asked to pay her frequent visits (2) and perhaps take her out for a short while (1).

She should be encouraged to keep herself clean with help from the nurses (2). Attention to her bowels may be needed as the elderly frequently worry about constipation (2); mild laxatives may be ordered by the doctor (1).

Any physical defect will be diagnosed and treatment ordered by the doctors

(2). New teeth or spectacles may be needed in order to help her lead as full a life as possible (2). She may need help with walking (2) and a physiotherapist may teach her to use a walking frame or stick (2).

In time the patient may be able to go home or to suitable residential accommodation (1).

(b) *Her diet* (25 marks)

Patients with malnutrition are often unwilling to eat as they may have been without proper food for some time (1). At first, highly nourishing drinks should be given every two hours (2) such as soups, flavoured Complan, flavoured or plain milk, Benger's food, Marmite, Bovril (3 for any 3 suggestions). Some elderly people will not drink anything cold and dislike plain water, whereas they may drink any amount of tea or orange juice (2). To encourage her to take an intake of 2—3 litres every 24 hours (2) she should be given whatever she will take and sugar can be added for extra calories (2).

As soon as possible more solid food should be added, especially foods which contain protein (2) such as fish, meat, eggs and cheese (2 for any 2).

Fruit which contains vitamin C must be given, such as oranges, lemons, grapefruit or tomatoes (2 for any 2).

To prevent constipation, roughage should be given (1), such as wholemeal bread or vegetables (1) which should be sieved at first (1).

The patient should be weighed at two- or three-day intervals (1) so that her progress can be assessed (1). Dietary supplements such as vitamins or iron are given as prescribed (2).

Geriatric Nursing

15 REHABILITATION AFTER AMPUTATION OF THE LEG

REVISION QUIZ

In each of questions 1–6 there is only ONE correct answer. You have to choose this; so write A, B or C, etc., ONLY.

1. An elderly man has just been transferred from a surgical ward, where he had a below knee amputation, to the geriatric assessment unit. He has no one at home to look after him. Is the main purpose of a geriatric assessment unit

   A. to give nursing care to patients who cannot be discharged from hospital
   B. to act as a half-way house until they can be admitted to an old people's home
   C. to rehabilitate them and decide what help they are going to need

2. This patient has to learn how to put on and take off his new artificial leg. Would you

   A. leave this entirely to the physiotherapist
   B. ask if you can be there while the physiotherapist shows him
   C. examine the leg so that you can show him yourself

3. Soon after his arrival, he feels uncertain about getting to the lavatory. Would you

   A. help him to walk there
   B. give him a walking stick and show him where to go on his own
   C. wheel him there in a sani-chair
   D. give him a urinal

4. He finds it difficult to get out of bed and to dress himself, because his balance is not very certain. Would you

   A. let him sit on the bed and put his clothes on for him
   B. tell him he must learn and leave him to it
   C. stay with him but get him to do it on his own

5. This patient is a keen gardener and has been telling you about his garden and greenhouse. Should you

    A. explain that he will not be able to do gardening any more and suggest other interest such as handicrafts
    B. suggest other interests without telling him he won't be able to garden
    C. change the subject
    D. encourage him to think and talk about his garden

6. He tells you that he is worried about three steps to the bathroom in his home which have no hand-rail. Would you

    A. mention this to the hospital social worker
    B. mention it to the physiotherapist
    C. tell him that by the time he goes home he won't need a hand-rail
    D. tell him that the Local Authority Social Services Department will see to it when he gets home
    E. tell him not to worry as he will probably be rehoused in a flat

Now WRITE answers to the following questions.

7. A case conference is to be held in the unit to discuss the patient's rehabilitation and the help he is going to need in future. List any contributions which *you* might be able to make to this discussion.

8. List the people who may attend the case conference, and any who may have to be consulted even if they cannot attend it.

Now correct your answers from the notes on pages 109 and 110.

ANSWERS AND NOTES ON REVISION QUIZ

For questions 1–6 count TWO marks for each correct answer

Correct answer

1. C. To rehabilitate each patient as far as possible, and to consider what
        help they will need after discharge—and whether they can go
        home, or need some other form of accommodation.

2. B. Teaching the patient how to manage his artificial limb will really be
        the job of the surgical appliance fitter and the physiotherapist. But
        you should find out what they have told him, as there will be many
        occasions when a physiotherapist won't be there if he gets into
        difficulties.

3. A. You have to make the patient as independent as possible; but he
4. C. will need help in this. He should get into the habit of walking and
        looking after himself; but may need encouragement to give him
        confidence.

5. D. There is no real reason why he should not be able to do gardening if his rehabilitation is successful. Talking and thinking about it will encourage him to persevere.

6. A. Minor adjustments in the house should be done before the patient goes home. The hospital social worker can contact the Social Services Department; or she may be able to get the patient's son or son-in-law to do it.

For questions 7 and 8 count marks as indicated.

7. You should be able to report how independent the patient has become in such things as getting in and out of bed, washing and dressing himself, getting into the bath, etc. (1 mark for each = 3).

    You might need to mention his interests, such as garden or workshop (1). These would be a strong argument for getting him back to his own home, rather than to a flat or old people's home where he could not pursue them (1). Where he is going to live will be one of the main things the conference has to discuss.

    Any worries, especially about small things, which the patient has told you (1). He may have been diffident about mentioning them to the doctor, or not have thought of them at the time.

8. The surgeon who did his operation (1); the consultant in the geriatric unit (1); the nursing staff (1); physiotherapist (1); hospital social worker (1); surgical appliance fitter (1). People who will be responsible for helping him in the community may also be there, or should at least be consulted: his own general practitioner (1), health visitor (1) and district nurse attached to the practice (1); social workers in the community (1); home help superintendent (1).

Maximum Total = 29 marks.

Your score will show you how well you have done. Do any more revision which you think you need BEFORE attempting the question on the page opposite.

QUESTION

Without looking back or consulting any book, write the answer to the question on this page. You should not take more than 40 minutes to plan and write your answer.

An elderly widower who cannot yet go home following a below-knee amputation has been transferred to a geriatric unit.

(a) List the members of the caring team who will be involved in assessing his needs and helping with his rehabilitation.

(b) What part will you play in the rehabilitation of this patient?

When you have finished your answer, and not before, turn over and correct it by the 'model answer' overleaf.

MODEL ANSWER

(a) *The caring team* (30 marks)

The orthopaedic surgeon (*or* surgeon who did the operation)
The geriatric consultant
Nursing staff
Physiotherapists
Hospital social worker
Surgical appliance fitter
The patient's general practitioner
Health visitor
Social workers in the community
District nurse
Home help (*or* Home help supervisor)

Count 3 marks each for any 10 = 30 marks.

(b) *The nurse's part in rehabilitation* (70 marks)

As nurses see more of the patients than other members of the team (3), I should have many opportunities of encouraging this patient (4). When the physiotherapists are not there he will need encouragement and help in walking (2), doing his exercises (2) and trying to cope with stairs (2).

I should encourage him to do as much as he could for himself (4), and not be too dependent on the nurses (2). I should give any necessary help (2), but try to make him independent in getting in and out of bed (2), putting on and taking off his artificial leg (2), dressing himself (2) and getting in and out of the bath (2). I would praise his successes in doing these things (2).

I might be able also to get him to think of ways in which he could help himself in his own home (3). I would encourage him to discuss these ideas with his grown up children, if he had any (3), as they might be able to help by doing small things such as fixing up hand-rails in his house (2 for this or any other example).

I would also encourage him to talk about his hobbies and interests at home (4), and to believe that he will be able to take them up again (3), as this will help him to persevere in his rehabilitation (3).

When there was a case conference to discuss his needs, I should be able to report on how independent he was now (4). It might be important to report what he had told me about his interests (3). For example, if his main interest were his garden or workshop, it would be important that he should not be rehoused in a flat with no opportunities for going on with his hobbies (3). He might also have told me about small worries which he had not liked to mention to the doctors or social worker (2).

Patients do not always remember or quite understand all that they are told by doctors, social workers, etc.; if necessary I would explain anything of this kind which the patient was worried about (2); or ask the doctor or social worker to explain it to him again (3). In these ways I would try to show him that the whole team was working together (2), and to reassure him that he would get the help he needed when he went home (2).

Geriatric Nursing

16 THE ELDERLY CONFUSED PATIENT

REVISION QUIZ

In each of questions 1–5 there is only ONE correct answer. You have to choose this; so write A, B or C, etc., ONLY.

1. Mrs Barker is an elderly patient just admitted to your ward. She is obviously confused and disorientated. You find twelve £1 notes in her handbag. Should you

   A. put the handbag in her locker and tell her to look after it
   B. give the handbag to her daughter and ask her to take it home
   C. give the notes to her daughter, asking her to sign a receipt, and leave the handbag with Mrs Barker
   D. check the money with another nurse, enter it in the ward property book and take it to the Secretary's office

2. If there is a choice, would you give Mrs Barker a bed

   A. in a side ward with two other patients
   B. at the far end of the main ward
   C. near the door in the main ward
   D. in the centre of the main ward

3. Mrs Barker is frail, but has been up and about at home. Do you consider that it would be best

   A. to nurse her in bed, with cot sides
   B. to nurse her in bed, without cot sides
   C. to let her be up most of the time, wearing her own clothes
   D. to let her be up in her nightdress and dressing gown

4. Her daughter visits her at tea-time the day after she is admitted. Would you

   A. ask her to leave the ward while her mother has her tea
   B. encourage her to help her mother herself while she has her tea
   C. feed the old lady and allow the daughter to stay

5. Mr John Robinson is also elderly and very confused. He has with him a pipe, tobacco and matches. Should you

    A. say that smoking is not allowed, and give the things to his relatives to take away with them

    B. leave the pipe, tobacco and matches with him

    C. tactfully remove the matches only, and tell him to ask if he wants to smoke

Now WRITE answers to the following questions.

6. List ways in which (a) nurses and (b) relatives can help a confused patient to retain a sense of who she is and of her own dignity.

7. List any measures nurses can take to prevent such patients (a) from becoming incontinent or (b) from disturbing the ward at night.

8. List the advantages of allowing confused elderly patients to be out of bed as much as possible during the day.

9. List any risks which must be considered in allowing them to be up and about.

Now correct your answers from the notes on pages 117 and 118.

ANSWERS AND NOTES ON REVISION QUIZ

For questions 1–5 count TWO marks for each correct answer.

Correct answer

1. C. A confused patient should obviously not have a lot of money with her, as this can get lost. On the other hand, there is no reason why she should be deprived of her handbag. As Mrs Barker has a relative with her, the money should be given to her; but she must give a receipt for it. Only if the patient has no relative with her should the money be kept in the hospital, as in D.

2. D. The centre of the ward is probably best. Nurses should be able to see the patient easily. If she is too near the door, she can more easily wander out of the ward.

3. C. If she is well enough, she should be up as much as possible, and wear her own clothes. Elderly patients can deteriorate physically and mentally if kept in bed. A confused patient may keep getting out of bed, and be liable to fall. She will feel more natural in her own clothes, and it will be easier for her to move about.

4. B. Relatives are usually pleased to do small things to help patients and it helps them to keep in contact.

5.   C.   He should not have matches, as confused patients do sometimes set their bedclothes on fire. But he may be very miserable if not allowed to smoke at all and separated from his pipe and tobacco. Someone should be with him if he smokes; this is another thing which relatives can help with if nurses are too busy.

For questions 6–9 count marks as indicated.

6.   (a)   Nurses should address patients by name as Mr, Mrs or Miss (1); listen to what they say and give reasonable answers (1); coax, not scold (1); in fact, treat them as people, even if they *are* confused.

     (b)   Frequent visiting is important (1); seeing familiar people helps the patient to keep in touch with her own life (1) and reassures her that she is not abandoned (1).

7.   (a)   Patients should have *regular* attention to sanitary needs every two hours (1), and more often if necessary (1). The may need showing more than once where the lavatory is if they are up and about (1).

     (b)   Nurses should see that patients have had bedpans or urinals before settling for the night (1) and that they are comfortable (1). There should be a shaded light over the bed; being in the dark may make them more confused (1).

8.   *Advantages*: the patient is not so likely to fall out of bed or get out and fall (1); feels more normal and freer (1); avoids complications such as hypostatic pneumonia (1) and bedsores (1).

9.   *Risks*: more risk of the patient wandering out of the ward (1); perhaps more likely to annoy other patients, e.g. by taking things from lockers (1).

Maximum Total = 28 marks.

Your score will show you how well you have done. Do any more revision which you think you need BEFORE attempting the question on the page opposite.

QUESTION

Without looking back or consulting any book, write the answer to the question on this page. You should not take more than 40 minutes to plan and write your answer.

Describe the main points in the nursing care of elderly confused patients. How can relatives and friends help?

When you have finished your answer, and not before, turn over and correct it by the 'model answer' overleaf.

MODEL ANSWER

Nursing care (75 marks)

If well enough, elderly confused patients should be up and dressed for as much of the day as possible (6). They feel less imprisoned and more natural than if they were kept in bed (2); and if in bed they may be continually getting out and may fall (2). Being up will also help to prevent complications such as hypostatic pneumonia (3) and bedsores (3), and will probably lead to their sleeping better at night (2).

These patients have to be watched to make sure they do not wander out of the ward (4), or steal from other patients' lockers (2). They should not have any matches (2), and if they want to smoke someone must be with them (3).

Nurses should talk to them reasonably, and coax them rather than scolding them (3). Addressing them by name as Mrs, Mr or Miss helps them to keep a sense of their own identity and dignity (3).

Any valuables or considerable sums of money should be taken home by relatives (4), and signed for by them (2). If there are no relatives, valuables must be entered in the ward property book (2), signed for by two nurses (2), and taken to the hospital secretary's office for safekeeping (2).

Nurses will have to make sure that these patients eat their meals (3), and especially that they drink enough (3). They will also need help with washing and dressing, so that they are kept clean and tidy (3).

Regular attention to their sanitary needs is necessary to prevent incontinence (5). They should be taken to the lavatory, or use a commode, every two hours (2).

The bed of a confused patient should be in a position in which it can easily be seen by the nurses both by day and night (5). At night there should be a shaded light over it (3), as being in the dark often makes patients more confused (2). Cot sides may be necessary at night (2).

How relatives and friends can help (25 marks)

By visiting frequently relatives and friends can help a patient to keep in touch with reality (5). She is reassured by seeing familiar faces (2), and does not feel so abandoned (2).

Visitors can do many small things for the patient which the nurses may not have time for (2), such as finding things in her locker (2), sitting and talking to her (2) or sitting with a patient who wants to smoke (2). They can take her for a little walk round the ward if she is restless (2); can help her with her meals (2), and with washing and doing her hair (2). They can also brighten her life by bringing in things she likes to eat, provided these are allowed (2).

Geriatric Nursing

17 FRACTURE OF THE FEMUR

REVISION QUIZ

A fracture of the femur in an elderly person is usually in the region of the neck of the femur. Generally it is repaired by means of a 'pin' or 'pin and plate', as shown below.

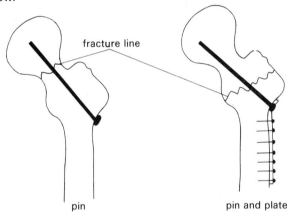

fracture line

pin   pin and plate

The object of this treatment is to allow the patient to get up and start rehabilitation as soon as possible, thus avoiding the many complications which can occur if he or she is kept in bed. The *nursing* consists in helping with this early rehabilitation and preventing the complications.

To revise this, make yourself a chart on a large sheet of paper, as follows:

Organs	Complications	Prevention	Observations
Lungs			
Urinary system			
Bowels			
Skin			
Joints, Muscles			
Circulation			
Brain			

The first column lists the main organs and systems which may be affected if an elderly person is confined to bed. You should fill in the other columns with a few words listing the complications, how they can be prevented by good nursing and the observations which the nurse should make.

Now correct your answers from the notes on pages 123 and 124.

ANSWERS AND NOTES ON REVISION QUIZ

Lungs (9 marks)

Complication: hypostatic pneumonia (2).

Prevention: encourage movement (1); get patient up (1); encourage breathing exercises (1).

Observations: note rise of temperature (1) and pulse (1); note respiration rate (1) and moist-sounding breathing (1).

Urinary system (9 marks)

Complications: cystitis and pyelitis (*or* urinary infection) (2); this may lead to stones in kidney (1) or to renal failure (1).

Prevention: sufficient fluid intake (1); prompt attention to sanitary needs so that patient is not afraid to drink (1).

Observations: fluid balance chart (1); observation for concentrated or cloudy urine (1) or rise of temperature (1).

Bowels (8 marks)

Complications: constipation (2); impacted faeces (2).

Prevention: roughage in diet (1); sufficient fluid intake (1); aperients if necessary (1).

Observations: of bowel movements (1).

Skin (6 marks)

Complications: pressure sores (2).

Prevention: change of position in bed (1); getting up (1); routine treatment of pressure areas (1).

Observations: on condition of pressure areas (1).

Joints, muscles (10 marks)

Complications: contractures of joints (2), especially hips (1) and knees (1); muscle wasting (1).

Prevention: encourage to move (1) and do exercises (1); get up (1) and encourage to walk (1); patient should wear own shoes to make this easier (1).

Circulation (9 marks)

Complications: deep venous thrombosis (2); pulmonary embolus (2).

Prevention: encourage movement (1) and leg exercises (1); get patient to stand and walk (1).

Observations: of pain in legs (1); slight rise of temperature (1).

Brain (9 marks)

Complications: mental confusion (2); may lead to incontinence (2).

Prevention: keep up interest in surroundings (1); encourage visitors (1); encourage patient to help herself (1).

Observations: for signs of confusion (1) or apathy (1)

Maximum Total = 60 marks. You will have done very well if you scored 50 or more.

Spend a few minutes reading through the above and considering how it affects details of nursing care of a patient with a fracture of the femur.

Do any more revision which you think you need BEFORE attempting the question on the page opposite.

QUESTION

Without looking back or consulting any book, write the answer to the question on this page. You should not take more than 40 minutes to plan and write your answer.

An elderly patient falls and fractures a femur.

(a) What complications may occur as a result of being confined to bed?

(b) How can the nurse help with early ambulation and rehabilitation of this patient?

When you have finished your answer, and not before, turn over and correct it by the 'model answer' overleaf.

MODEL ANSWER

(a) *Complications resulting from being confined to bed* (40 marks)

Hypostatic pneumonia (*or* chest infection) (5).

Cystitis and pyelitis (*or* urinary infection) (4); this can lead to renal failure (2) or stones in the kidney (1).

Constipation (3) and impacted faeces (2).

Pressure sores (4), especially on sacrum (1) and heels (1).

Incontinence (3).

Mental confusion (3).

Contractures of joints (3); dropped foot (2); wasting of muscles (1).

Thrombosis of leg veins (*or* deep venous thrombosis) (3), which may lead to a pulmonary embolus (2).

(b) *Early ambulation and rehabilitation* (60 marks)

At first the nurse helps the patient out of bed into a chair while the bed is made (2), supporting her so that she gains confidence (2). She should be helped to dress so that she feels more normal (3), and should wear her own shoes so that standing and walking are easier (3). She should be out of bed as much as possible (2), but the nurse must see that she does not get too tired (2) or cold (2). She must be helped to move and her pressure areas must be attended to so that they do not get sore from sitting in a chair (3). The nurse must encourage her to do leg exercises (1) and breathing exercises (1) which the physiotherapist has taught her. She should be encouraged to wash herself, but given any help necessary (2).

When the patient starts to walk on crutches or with a stick, the nurse must be ready to help her so that she gets as much practice as possible (5).

The nurse should also encourage her to eat well (3), making sure that she can reach her food (2). She should be given some fruit or other food containing roughage to prevent constipation (2); and she must drink enough (3) to prevent urinary infection (2).

She must be helped to use a commode, or taken to the lavatory in a sani-chair (2) as often as she requires it (2); otherwise she may be afraid to drink enough (2) or become incontinent (1). The nurse must notice if she is becoming constipated (3), as she may need an aperient (1); if she is reluctant to drink it is necessary to keep a fluid balance chart (2).

She should be encouraged to take an interest in what is going on around her (2), and in her own appearance (2). Visitors should be welcomed (2), so that she keeps up her interest in life at home (1).

Geriatric Nursing

18 TERMINAL NURSING CARE

REVISION QUIZ

For questions 1–4 there is only ONE correct answer. You have to choose this; then write A, B or C, etc., ONLY.

1. Mr Andrews is to be admitted for nursing care as he lives alone. He has a terminal illness, but at the time of admission is well enough to get up when he feels able to do so. Where would be the most suitable place in the ward for his bed

    A. in the ward where he can see and talk to other patients
    B. in a corner of the ward with the curtains drawn
    C. in a side-room
    D. in the ward at first, then in a side-room if he wished

2. Should Mr Andrew's elderly sister be allowed to

    A. visit him whenever she likes for as long as she can
    B. stay as long as she can and help with his care
    C. visit during visiting hours only, at first
    D. come when she likes but leave whenever any care is needed by the patient

3. While Mr Andrews is well enough, should he be

    A. kept up all day in his nightclothes
    B. kept up all day dressed in his day clothes
    C. kept in bed and allowed up for bedmaking and toilet purposes
    D. allowed to please himself

4. If Mr Andrews is in pain, would you

    A. Check to see whether he had had any drugs during the last four hours and only ask for a further dose if he had not
    B. consult his drug-sheet to see if he were prescribed a drug for 'whenever required' so he could have another dose
    C. try and make him comfortable without the aid of drugs and explain that he only had his dose four hours ago

D. make him a hot drink, change his position but tell him he cannot have any more drugs for the time being

Now WRITE answers to the following question.

5. List how the following people can help in Mr Andrews' care:

    (a) the chaplain
    (b) the dietician
    (c) the social worker

Now correct your answers from the notes on pages 129 and 130.

ANSWERS AND NOTES ON REVISION QUIZ

For questions 1–4 count TWO marks for each correct answer.

Correct answer

1. D. In the last stages of a terminal illness, some patients do prefer the quiet of a side-ward; there should be no hard and fast rule about this: some patients like company and dislike being 'shut away' or may be afraid of being left alone. As this patient lived alone, he might appreciate the company of the other patients. Also, if the patient were put into a side-ward on admission, he might feel that this was the 'last stage' in his illness.

2. B. There are many things this patient's sister may like to do for him and she will derive much comfort from being able to do so. As she is also elderly, she should not be allowed to become tired and should not be made to feel she has to stay and help care for her brother.

3. D. This may vary from day to day; these patients should be encouraged to get up and dress, but on the days when they do not feel so well, they should not be forced or made to feel they are not cooperating.

4. B. Drugs should never be withheld if they are needed by patients with a terminal illness. Pain is sometimes very severe and constant pain is tiring and depressing. Even drugs of addiction should be given as often as prescribed and doctors would want to know if the patient needs more than they have written up for him.

For question 5 count marks as indicated.

5. (a) Will be able to talk freely about death if the patient wishes (2). Will be able to reassure the patient and help remove fear (2). Bringing Communion (*or* Last Rites) to the patient will give comfort (2). Relatives may also be comforted if they know the patient's spiritual welfare is being catered for (2). This will depend if the patient has religious beliefs and welcomes visits from the chaplain.

   (b) Will find out the patient's food preferences so he can be given food and drinks that he enjoys, if possible (2). May be able to advise staff on suitable food or drink if the patient can only tolerate fluids or semi-solids (2). May be able to order special food or drink for him (2).

   (c) Will be able to alleviate any problems regarding property, rent payments or other home commitments (2). May be able to get in touch with relatives (2). Will be able to arrange for his pension to be collected (2). Will be able to assist financially if relatives cannot afford fare to visit the patient (2). May be able to arrange for patient to go home, or to relatives, for a day or two if he is well enough (2).

Possible total = 24 marks.

Maximum Total = 32 marks.

Your score will show you how well you have done. Do any more revision which you think you need BEFORE attempting the question on the page opposite.

QUESTION

Without looking back or consulting any book, write the answer to the question on this page. You should not take more than 40 minutes to plan and write your answer.

You are caring for an elderly female patient who is dying. What special care will your patient need? What are your responsibilities to the relatives of this patient?

When you have finished your answer, and not before, turn over and correct it by the 'model answer' overleaf.

MODEL ANSWER

Items arranged under headings for easy correcting; 100 marks are allowed.

Freedom from pain. Analgesics should be given as often as required, according to the doctor's prescription (10).

Physical comfort should be maintained with a well-made bed free from creases and crumbs (4). Clean linen should be used whenever needed (2). The patient's position should be changed two-hourly to prevent pressure sores (4) and the skin over the pressure areas kept clean and dry (4).

Baths should be given daily: in the bathroom for as long as possible, later in bed (3); hands and face are washed after meals (2).

The mouth should be kept moist and fresh and dentures cleaned after food and last thing at night (5).

Her hair should look as attractive as possible, being washed every two or three weeks (*or* she should be visited by the hairdresser) (3).

Her nails should be kept well-groomed (2).

Nightwear should be clean and as attractive as possible when she is confined to bed; if she is up, she should be encouraged to dress in comfortable clothes (5).

Food and drink should be attractively served, offered in small helpings as she fancies (5). If she has to be fed, the nurse should not appear in a hurry (2) and should flavour the food as the patient likes (2).

Drinks should be given frequently according to taste (3).

Relatives may like to bring small luxury foods from home and these can be encouraged if the patient enjoys it (2).

Urinary output should be observed and if the patient is incontinent she should be attended to at once (3).

Bowels. Mild laxatives or suppositories may be ordered to avoid straining; medication may also be ordered if there is diarrhoea (3). As long as possible, the patient should be taken or helped to the lavatory or lifted onto a commode for comfort (2).

Occupation. The patient may like to read, listen to the radio, watch television or play card games with other patients, even for short periods (4). A change of scene is often enjoyed so her bed or chair may be moved near a different window or she may be taken into the garden (3). Relatives may be able to take her out or even home for the day or a weekend with support from her general practitioner (3).

Spiritual comfort from the hospital chaplain or her parish priest may be desired and he will visit as often as possible (4). If she wishes to talk about her death, the nurse must show herself ready to listen and give reassurance that she will not be left alone (3).

Relatives and friends should be made welcome and allowed to visit often so the patient does not lose touch with the world outside the hospital (4). They can be encouraged to help with her care (*or* can help feed, wash, read to her) (3).

They may need support from the social worker or chaplain (2). They can be advised to go to their general practitioner if they are not sleeping (2).

They should be offered tea or coffee when it is served in the ward (2).

If they wish, the sister will arrange for them to see the consultant about the patient (2). Nursing staff can often give comfort and answer questions (2).

First Aid and Emergencies

19 FIRE! FIRE!

REVISION QUIZ

1. During your training you will have attended lectures from officers of the fire brigade. Write a list of as many things as you can remember which they talked about or demonstrated.

2. What arrangements must be made in any large building in order to protect the occupants from fire?

3. Write down any fire risks which apply especially to hospitals, and how patients are protected from them.

4. Do you know the positions of the fire extinguishers and fire escapes which should be used if there is a fire in the ward in which you are working? If you are not certain, find out now.

In each of questions 5–8 there is only ONE correct answer. You have to choose this; so write A, B, or C, etc., ONLY.

5. In dealing with bed clothes on a patient's bed which were on fire, would you *first*

    A. pour water on them
    B. run for a fire extinguisher
    C. roll them up and stamp on them
    D. throw them out of the window
    E. ring the switchboard to alert the fire brigade

6. If a patient's nightdress was on fire would you

    A. lay her on the floor with the flames uppermost and cover with a blanket
    B. lay her on the floor with the flames underneath her and cover with a blanket
    C. pour cold water over the flames
    D. use a fire extinguisher

7. In case of a fire in the ward, should you

    A. shut all windows and open the ward doors
    B. shut all windows and keep the doors shut
    C. open doors and windows

8. For a patient with a burn of the arm and hand, would the correct first aid treatment, before sending for the doctor, be

    A. to give some aspirin
    B. to give some hot sweet tea
    C. to immerse the arm in a bowl of cold water
    D. to wrap the arm in sterile towels
    E. to lay up a dressing trolley and apply sterile tulle gras to the burn

Now correct your answers from the notes on pages 137 and 138.

ANSWERS AND NOTES ON REVISION QUIZ

For questions 1–4 count marks as indicated.

1. The main subjects should be: care in preventing fires (1); preventing fires spreading by excluding air (1) (*or* examples such as closing doors and windows); extinguishers used for different kinds of fire and how to use them (1); extinguishing fires by excluding air (*or* examples such as dealing with clothing on fire) (1); methods of moving patients out of danger (1); use of fire escapes (1); how to contact the fire brigade (1).

   Possible total = 7 marks.

2. There must be fire doors (1) which are always kept shut (1); fire alarms (1); fire escapes (1); fire drills (1); officers of the fire brigade inspect to see that arrangements are satisfactory (1).

   Possible total = 6 marks.

3. Special dangers in hospitals are the use of oxygen (1); explosive gases in theatres (1); static electricity in theatres (1). Patients are protected by forbidding smoking etc. where oxygen is used (1), earthing trolleys and other apparatus in theatres (1) and avoiding use of nylon clothing in theatres (1).

   Possible total = 6 marks.

4. Count 3 marks if you are able to say where extinguishers and fire escapes are situated.

For questions 5–8 count TWO marks for each correct answer.

Correct answer

5. C. Exclude air by rolling up bedclothes with flames inside. This is the immediate action; fire extinguisher can be used later if clothes are still smouldering. The fire brigade must also be informed.

6. A. Flames must be uppermost, otherwise they will cause the whole body to be burnt. Cover with a blanket to exclude air and beat out the flames.

7. B. Shut all doors and windows to exclude air and prevent draughts which fan the flames.

8. C. Immerse the arm in cold water to take heat out of the burn as quickly as possible. In hospital, where you can get a doctor quickly, nothing else would be needed before he came.

Maximum Total = 30 marks.

Your score will show you how well you have done. Do any more revision which you think you need BEFORE attempting the question on the page opposite.

QUESTION

Without looking back or consulting any book, write the answer to the question on this page. You should not take more than 40 minutes to plan and write your answer.

What measures are taken in hospital to protect patients from the risk of fire?

You observe that a patient's bed-clothes are on fire.

(a) What immediate action would you take?
(b) Describe the first-aid treatment you would give to this patient who has burns on his right arm.

(*Hint to the student.* Notice that there are *three* parts to this question. Don't make the mistake of leaving out the first part and starting with (a).)

When you have finished your answer, and not before, turn over and correct it by the 'model answer' overleaf.

MODEL ANSWER

Measures to protect patients (50 marks)

There are fire doors throughout the hospital (3), which must be kept closed (3). There are also fire alarms (2), extinguishers (2) and escapes (2); instructions 'In case of fire' are displayed in every department (2). Staff are trained in using extinguishers (2) and fire practices are held (2).

Officers of the fire brigade inspect to make sure precautions are satisfactory (3). They also give talks and demonstrations regularly (3) to all members of the staff (2). These deal with fire prevention (2), preventing fires spreading (2), dealing with clothing on fire (2), the use of fire-fighting apparatus (2) and methods of moving patients out of danger (5). Staff are also taught the procedure for contacting the fire brigade (3).

Smoking and naked lights are forbidden (2) where there are explosive gases or oxygen (2). Danger from static electricity in theatres is prevented by earthing trolleys (2) and avoiding use of nylon clothing (2).

Bedclothes on fire (50 marks)

Immediate action. I would roll up the bedclothes with the flames on the inside (5) and try to extinguish them by stamping on or beating them (3). I would call to anyone near by to close windows (5), to get the nearest extinguisher (3) and to inform the person in charge of the ward (2), who would ring the switchboard so that the fire brigade would be informed (3).

I would try to reassure the patients so that there was no panic (5). Wheels of beds could be wound down in case it was necessary to move them away from the fire (2), and ambulant patients helped to another part of the ward or into the day-room (2).

First-aid treatment. I would fetch a bowl of cold water and immerse the burnt arm in it (5). The patient should be seated in an arm-chair (2), or put in an empty bed (1). If he is able to get up he could sit by the ward wash-basin with water running over his arm (4). He should be reassured (2) and told that a doctor will be coming as soon as possible (2). The person in charge will send for a doctor (3), and in the meantime the patient should have nothing by mouth (1).

First Aid and Emergencies

20 FRACTURED CLAVICLE; CUT HAND; BLEEDING VARICOSE VEIN; FOREIGN BODY IN NOSE

REVISION QUIZ

In each of the following questions there is only ONE correct answer. You have to choose this, so write A, B, or C, etc., ONLY.

1. If you believed that a child had a fractured clavicle, would you

    A. improvise a large arm sling
    B. improvise a collar-and-cuff sling
    C. improvise a St John's (or triangular sling)
    D. keep the arm straight and tie it to the body

2. Would you give this child

    A. some hot sweet tea   B. some hot milk
    C. some fruit juice   D. whichever he liked
    E. nothing by mouth

3. The hospital is a quarter of a mile away. Will this child

    A. need an ambulance   B. be able to walk there

4. A young girl has a deep cut in the palm of her hand caused by broken glass. Should you first

    A. elevate her arm   B. rest it on a table
    C. allow it to hang by her side

5. In treating the cut, should you

    A. put a tourniquet round her wrist
    B. put a tourniquet round her upper arm
    C. apply pressure with a dressing bandaged on firmly
    D. apply a dressing and bandage it on lightly

6. Having treated the cut, would you put on

    A. a large arm sling   B. a small arm sling
    C. a St John's sling   D. a collar-and-cuff sling

7. This girl feels faint. Should you give her

    A. a glass of water   B. a cup of hot tea
    C. some brandy   D. nothing by mouth

8. An elderly woman is bleeding from a ruptured varicose vein. Should you

    A. sit her in an armchair
    B. sit her in an armchair with the bleeding leg on another chair
    C. lay her flat and elevate the leg

9. Should you

    A. apply a tourniquet to this woman's leg
    B. apply a dressing with a firm bandage
    C. bandage it lightly

10. May this patient

    A. have a cup of tea   B. have nothing by mouth

11. A child pushes a small hard object up his nose. Should you

    A. try to get it out with a bodkin
    B. leave it alone and take him to the doctor
    C. give him pepper and make him sneeze

12. Would you give this child

    A. a glass of hot milk   B. a drink of fruit juice
    C. a packet of crisps   D. nothing by mouth

Now correct your answers from the notes on pages 143 and 144.

ANSWERS AND NOTES ON REVISION QUIZ

Count TWO marks for each correct answer.

Correct answer

1. C. The object is to keep the *elbow* supported, as this relieves pain. The clavicle is part of the shoulder girdle, to which the arm is attached. If the arm hangs it drags on the fractured clavicle and causes pain. A St John's sling supports the elbow and takes the weight of the arm. As a temporary measure, the patient can support his own elbow with his other hand, or it can be rested on a table.

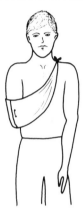

2. E. It might be safest to give nothing by mouth. If he only has a fractured clavicle he probably will not be having a general anaesthetic. But you could have made the wrong diagnosis and if he had, say, a fractured humerus or shoulder injury, he might need a general anaesthetic.

3. B. He should be able to walk, especially as it is not far.

4. A. Elevate the arm. Deep cuts in the palm of the hand bleed a lot. Elevating the arm slows up the bleeding.

5. D. You do not apply pressure to the wound as there may be bits of glass in it, and this may cause them to pierce more blood vessels. You put on a clean dressing and bandage lightly, relying on keeping the hand elevated to arrest the bleeding. Tourniquets are dangerous, and quite unnecessary for this kind of injury.

6.   C.   A St John's sling is best for keeping the hand elevated (see above).

7.   A.   She will probably not need a general anaesthetic, but again she *might*. But a glass of water will not do much harm, and she will probably need it if she feels faint. It might be best to restrict her intake to sips of water.

8.   C.   Lay her flat, and elevate the leg as high as possible. Varicose veins are stretched and dilated, so blood has pooled up above the bleeding point, and pours out from above. You should raise the leg above the level of the heart, so that it is helped to return to the heart. This usually stops the bleeding quite quickly.

9.   B.   Apply a dressing with a firm bandage. This helps to close up the dilated vein. Applying a tourniquet is the *worst* thing you can do, as it prevents blood from returning to the heart.

10.   A.   *This* patient will *not* have surgery, so there is no question of her having a general anaesthetic.

11.   B.   Leave it alone and take the child straight to the doctor. The danger is that the child will inhale the object; it then may stick in his larynx and cause asphyxia, or cause a lung abscess. There is great danger of pushing it further up if you poke anything up the nose. He is more likely to inhale if he cries or screams, as he may well do if you do anything drastic, so everyone should keep calm.

12.   D.   This child is practically certain to have a general anaesthetic while he has the foreign body removed. Without one he is almost certain to struggle and scream, making the procedure dangerous. So he should be given nothing by mouth.

Maximum Total = 24 marks.

Your score will show you how well you have done. Do any more revision which you think you need BEFORE attempting the question on the page opposite.

QUESTION

Without looking back or consulting any book, write the answer to the question on this page. You should not take more than 40 minutes to plan and write your answer.

Give a brief account of the action you would take in the following emergencies.

(a) A child falls off a swing and you believe he has fractured his clavicle (collar bone).

(b) Your friend cuts her hand when she stumbles near a window and puts her hand through the glass.

(c) A woman in a shop knocks her leg against a trolley and starts to bleed profusely from a varicose vein.

(d) A small child has pushed a bead up his nose.

(*Hints to the student:* In this sort of question you have to use your imagination and think what first aid treatment you *could* do, say, in a park or a shop or wherever the accident occurs. You have to deal with the emergency as a whole, not just treat the patient. Don't forget that children have mothers!)

When you have finished your answer, and not before, turn over and correct it by the 'model answer' overleaf.

MODEL ANSWER

(a) *Fractured clavicle* (25 marks)

I would try to comfort the child (2), and find somewhere for him to sit down (2). I would get him to support the elbow on the injured side with his other hand (4), as this will help to relieve the pain (1). If he is not near home I would then improvise a sling to support the elbow (4), and take him home (2). If he is in his own garden, the sling could be improvised in the house (1) while he rested his forearm on a table (1). The sling should be a St John's (*or* triangular) sling (3). I would advise his mother to take him to hospital (*or* to a doctor) as soon as possible (3), and say that he had better not have anything to eat or drink just in case his injury makes it necessary to have a general anaesthetic (2).

(b) *Hand cut on glass* (25 marks)

I would elevate the hand to lessen bleeding (3), and get my friend to sit down (2). If there was no sterile dressing available, I would apply a temporary dressing such as a clean piece of sheet or towel or a large clean handkerchief (2 for any ONE). I would bandage this on lightly (3), in case there was any glass in the wound (1). I would not try to remove pieces of glass, as this might increase bleeding (3). It would apply a St John's (*or* triangular) sling to keep the hand elevated (3). If my friend felt faint, I would get her to sit with her head between her knees (2) and she could have a glass of water (2), but she should not have anything else to eat or drink in case her injury needs treating under a general anaesthetic (2). I would take her to hospital (*or* to a doctor) as soon as possible (2).

(c) *Bleeding varicose vein* (25 marks)

I would ask one of the shop assistants to help me take this woman as quickly as possible somewhere where she can lie down (3), and then raise her leg as high as possible (*or* above the level of the heart) by holding it up (5) until the bleeding lessened (2). I would remove or loosen anything tight around her leg or waist (2). Possibly the shop would have some first-aid equipment; if so a clean pad should be put over the bleeding point (2) and bandaged on firmly (4). The woman could have a cup of tea if one was offered (2). If she had a husband or friend waiting outside, I would ask someone to fetch them (1), and advise them to take her to her doctor if they had a car (1). If not, or if she was alone, I would ask someone to ring for an ambulance (3).

(d) *Bead pushed up nose* (25 marks)

I would take it calmly and not frighten the child (3), and ask the mother to do the same and not to scold him (2), as he is more likely to inhale the bead if he cries or screams (3). I would get him to blow his nose (3), but if the bead did not come out easily, nothing should be poked up the nose (5). I would take him to hospital (*or* to a doctor) as quickly as possible (2), with his mother (2). He should have nothing to eat or drink, as he may be given an anaesthetic when the bead is removed (5).